Susan 20.

There's nothing horsey about this book but you are one of my friends who saw me through the saga to get it published!

Sa

Formulas for Motherhood in a Chinese Hospital

Formulas for Motherhood in a Chinese Hospital

SUZANNE GOTTSCHANG

University of Michigan Press
Ann Arbor

Published in the United States of America by
The University of Michigan Press
Manufactured in the United States of America
♾ Printed on acid-free paper

2021 2020 2019 2018 4 3 2 1

A CIP catalog record for this book is available from the British Library.

ISBN 978-0-472-13075-7 (hardcover : alk. paper)
ISBN 978-0-472-12362-9 (e-book)

This book is dedicated to my grandmothers, Veronica Walsh Niewerth and Virginia Kelley Turner

Contents

Acknowledgments

There are always so many people to thank after writing a book. While most authors end with thanks to their families, I wish to put mine at the beginning. My parents, Karen Turner and Tom Gottschang, brought me to visit them in China in 1985, and at the time I never imagined that I would end up as an anthropologist of China. Their support—intellectual, financial, and emotional—has made my work possible. They have been inspirations to me—my father for his commitment to using his expertise in economics for teaching, research, and collaboration with his colleagues in China and Vietnam, my mother for her cutting edge scholarship on early Chinese law and Vietnamese women soldiers. Their accomplishments notwithstanding, I have learned most from their strength, tenacity, intelligence, sense of humor, and love. My husband, Daniel Guidera, has seen me through the ups and downs of writing a book, and his love, advice, guidance, and sense of humor sustained me as I navigated the process of bringing this book to completion. My sister Kelley Gottschang, my sister-in-law Michele Meissner, and my nephew Drew Gottschang have always provided wonderful and fun distractions from writing. My four-legged family members, while they could not read or comment on drafts, kept me company, got me outdoors, and reminded me of the importance of living in the moment.

My interest in infant feeding came out of a class on maternal and child nutrition taught by Derrick and Patrice Jelliffe that I attended while I was studying for my masters in public health at the University of California, Los Angeles. Derrick Jelliffe would regularly remind the class that culture is not a black box when it comes to nutrition and food. At UCLA my first doctoral supervisor and mentor, Francesca Bray, now at the University of Edinburgh, provided support and direction, as well as friendship and inspiration, that continue to sustain me in my work. Rubie Watson, at the University of Pittsburgh, also mentored and guided me as I made my way from doctoral studies to fieldwork and through dissertation writing. Her longstanding friendship and support, along with that of Woody Watson at Harvard University, have contributed to the writing of this book. William Alford, director of the Harvard Law School's East Asian Legal Studies program, has provided me with an intellectual home at two different times in my career. Nancy Chen, Constance Clark, and Lyn Jeffrey were my partners in editing *China Urban* and helped me develop some of the threads of the argument presented in this book. Xiaodong Zhang, in Beijing and Worcester, Massachusetts, provided support and love during the uncertain times of fieldwork and dissertation writing. Wang Lihua's friendship, scholarship on Chinese women, and our conversations over these many years continues to sustain me. The Fairbank Center for East Asian Research at Harvard University granted me an An Wang post doctoral fellowship during which I had the time and space to expand and hone my ideas. My time at Harvard brought new colleagues into my life and provided an opportunity to renew old ones. In particular, the Gender Studies Workshop at the Fairbank Center, run by Christina Gilmartin and Ellen Widmer, provided me with the opportunity to try out my ideas and learn from other scholars in the field at their wonderful seminars and dinners. Further afield but no less important, Susan Greenhalgh has, from the moment I got up my nerve to introduce myself, been a friend and generous supporter of my work over these many years. Goncalo Santos, whose work in Guangdong Province brought us together at workshops at Manchester University, the Max Planck Institute, and the University of Hong Kong, has become a dear comrade in the study of reproduction in China.

In China the Academy of Preventive Medicine's Institute of Nutrition graciously arranged for my fieldwork in a local hospital. Its support and willingness to host a doctoral student made this research possible. Professor Dong Furen and his wife Dr. Liu Ainian, my Beijing "grandparents," took me for wonderful meals, included me in many holiday celebrations, and generally watched over me. Peter Gilmartin's friendship kept me in good coffee and conversation while conducting the research for this project. Christina Gilmartin was always ready to process fieldwork experiences and remained a good friend and colleague until her untimely death.

I want to thank my colleagues in anthropology at Smith College—Fernando Armstrong-Fumero, Elliot Fratkin, Donald Joralemon, Ravina Aggarwal, Elizabeth Hopkins, Pinky Hota, Elizabeth Klarich, and Caroline Melly—for their intellectual camaraderie and friendship. Lynn Morgan is a role model and friend who helped make this book possible. Nancy Cai helped at the last minute with formatting and the bibliography. J. Phillip Kistler made all this possible. This book would not have been completed without the ongoing support of Leslie King and Velma Garcia. Their friendship has meant more than I can say in an acknowledgment. My comrades from afar—Rachel Friedman, Alison Bianchi, and Ellen MacKay—are owed an immeasurable amount of gratitude for their support. My editor, Christopher Dreyer, along with Marcia LaBrenz at the University of Michigan Press have shepherded this book to its fruition and have made the process as painless as possible.

Funding for the research for this book includes a dissertation grant from the Committee on Scholarly Communications with China, an An Wang Postdoctoral Fellowship at Harvard University, a Picker Grant from Smith College, and faculty research grants from Smith College.

Finally, the women who allowed me into their lives, as well as the wonderful nurses and physicians at the hospital, made this book possible. I will always be grateful to them for including me in their lives at an intimate and important moment.

Note on Romanization: The Hanyu Pinyin system is used for romanization of the Chinese language.

Introduction

On the first day of my fieldwork in Beijing in 1994, Dr. Chang from the Ministry of Health's Institute of Nutrition climbed the front stairs of the Number 35 Hospital with me. As we reached the main entrance, she pointed to a brass placard with red Chinese characters and English letters and said, "This is a Baby-Friendly Hospital, and so this will be a good site for your research on infant feeding." The sign announced its mission and sponsors to patients and visitors: "A Baby Friendly Hospital (*Ai ying yi yuan*) under the aegis of China's Ministry of Public Health and the World Health Organization and United Nations Children's Fund." As we made our way to the obstetrics clinic, I was excited that I would be able to conduct research in a hospital that was participating in a global campaign to increase the number of breastfeeding mothers. In short, this initiative aims to reorganize hospital spaces and practices to encourage breastfeeding. What I discovered later is that China was, and continues to be, a leader in creating Baby-Friendly Hospitals (BFHs). One of over 4,500 BFHs certified through the mid-1990s, the Number 35 Hospital achieved its status by renovating clinics and maternity wards to accommodate breastfeeding education classes and rooming-in facilities for all mothers and infants during their hospital stay. This remarkable transformation of so many hospitals in China stands in contrast to other countries' participation in the initiative. For example, in 2014 the United States counted 198 hospitals certified as baby friendly by the United Nations Children's Fund UNICEF.[1]

Although I was most interested in how such a policy was put into operation, two posters in the Obstetrics clinic hallway brought home the variety of forces within and outside China that work to influence infant feeding practices. One, at the end of the hall on an unmarked door with frosted glass, depicted a chubby baby lying on its back, arms outstretched toward a flow of milk from a breast that appeared to be attached to a globe of the world (see fig. 1). The characters above the child on the poster read "Mama I want to drink [eat] milk (*mama wo yao chi nai* 妈妈我要吃奶]," and those to the right of the image read "Breastfeeding is Best (*muru weiyang hao* 母乳喂养好]." The door, though unmarked by other signage, also served as the entrance to the Number 35 Hospital's breastfeeding education room where pregnant women received instruction in the techniques and benefits of breastfeeding. Another poster made it clear that more than infant health was at stake in these corridors and clinic rooms. There, where nurses, doctors, and women addressed the practical realities of child bearing and nurturing, a poster's perfectly coiffed Asian woman, dressed in a negligee and pearls, held her infant, observed by a rather non-maternal-looking nurse. The text accompanying the image also proclaimed, "Breastfeeding Is Best." Yet the poster did not actually promote infant well-being; it advertised a Chinese medicinal tonic for restoring the mother's health after childbirth. The association of breastfeeding with a consumer product for mothers was a reminder that by the mid-1990s market socialism had established a presence in the realm of the hospital. Together, these images served as visual manifestations of the multilayered agendas surrounding infant feeding that extended from the hospital to the Chinese government and the international health community.

This book focuses on a group of urban women who navigated a path from pregnancy to motherhood and made decisions about how to feed their infants in a Beijing BFH. They did so during a

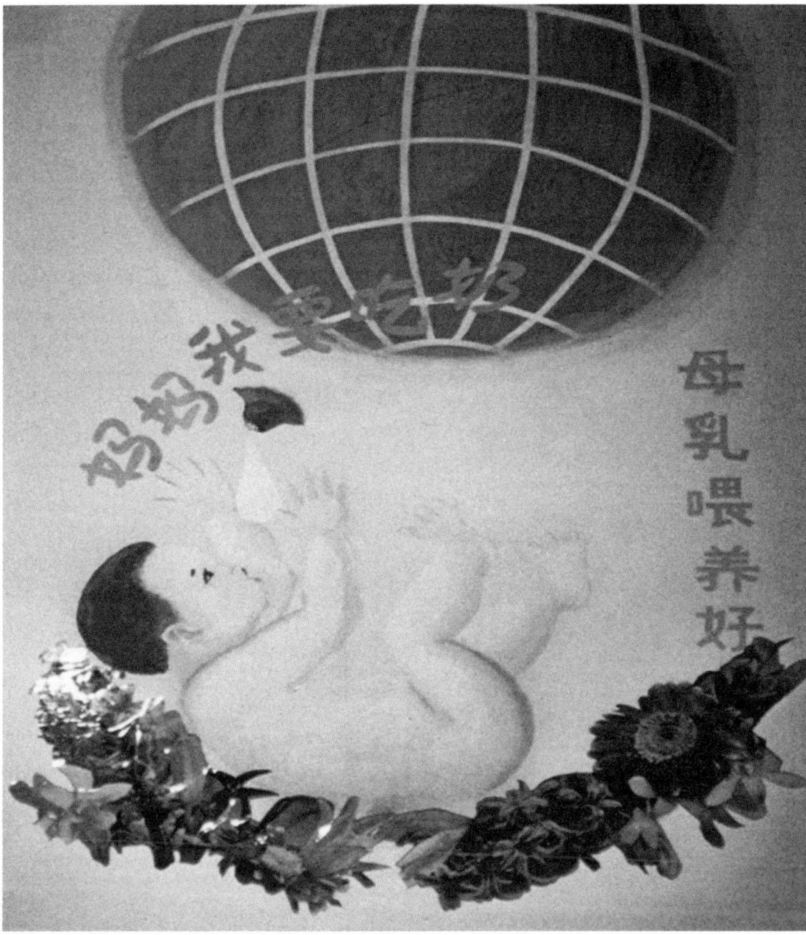

Figure 1. Poster in the hallway of the obstetrics clinic

time of extraordinary social, cultural, and economic change in China. As producers of healthy babies who would grow up to serve a modernizing nation-state, women could not escape the message that their decisions and practices resonated far beyond their households. Although the Chinese government did retreat from numerous policies that affected many aspects of life in the 1990s, in the realm of reproduction, the state, backed by the authority of multilateral bodies such as the World Health Organization (WHO), continued to exert pressure on women to conform to its directives. Yet urban Chinese mothers were also at the center of the social, cultural, and economic changes that brought foreign products such as infant formulas made by Nestle, Gerber's baby food, Pampers disposable diapers, and other infant care products to their local department stores. These products represented not only the opening of China's markets to foreign companies but also an expansion of ways to best nourish and care for children.[2] New mothers now faced a moment in their lives when decisions about how to feed their only children took on moral and individual importance with the availability of these new consumer products and a global maternal and child health policy promoting breastfeeding.[3] This book contributes to long-standing scholarship that helps to complicate our understandings of the ways in which individuals in China make decisions in the face of cultural pressures, family responsibilities, state policies, and global public health agendas.[4]

Global Health and Universal Mothers

> The lives of almost 1.5 million infants could be saved every year if for the first six months of life they were exclusively breastfed. (UNICEF 1997)

Breastfeeding, and infant feeding in general, may seem at first glance a rather narrow realm in which to examine the connections among motherhood, reproduction, and politics. After all it is only one of many practical aspects of rearing children. However, the goal of increasing breastfeeding among new mothers, especially in the global south, has served as a long-standing focus of the WHO's efforts to reduce infant disease and death in the last forty years. Medical and public health research attributes the worldwide decrease in breastfeeding to a variety of causes, including the availability of commercial infant formulas, urbanization, women's employment outside the home, and minimal or negative medical and social support.[5] In short, according to the WHO and a number of nongovernmental organizations (NGOs), potentially more than 1.5 million infant deaths a year could be prevented if all mothers in the world would breastfeed. Mothers, then, form the critical link in protecting children from death and disease. The poster of the infant suckling the breast/globe in figure 1 makes visible these connections. Producing healthy infants requires a commitment from mothers all over the world to breastfeed (Franklin, Lury, and Stacey 2000).

The connections among the actions of mothers, infant health, and the concerns of multilateral agencies, such as the WHO, that monitor and promote the health of the world's population represent a case of the workings of a form of biopolitics that extends beyond that of individual states.[6] Biopolitics operates in an organization like the WHO in the processes of defining health priorities, drafting regulations, and designing health programs aimed at solving widespread health problems. One aim of this book is to trace the connections between the biopolitics that underlie international- and national-level interests in infant feeding and the ways in which these reach mothers through their bodies and behaviors.[7] Infant feeding, then, offers a way to document how the cumulative effects of individual behavior become critical to the well-being of a population and indeed the world.[8] The epigraph that began this section exemplifies this logic: if every mother in the world breastfed her baby, then infants, as a group, would experience less illness and fewer deaths. At another level, documenting ideals and practices about motherhood promoted in a worldwide breastfeeding program allows us to see that public health, much like medicine, relies on the constitution of universal ideals of maternity and maternal bodies to bring about change (Ram and Jolly 1998).

Homing in on the lifesaving benefits of breastfeeding in dramatic and sweeping statements helps to justify and define the need for an international response. But in more specific ways, as programs like the Baby-Friendly Hospital Initiative (BFHI) are developed so are a variety of media (pamphlets, web pages, promotional posters) that outline their basic goals and structures. These media, in an effort to define the problems addressed by such global health initiatives as the BFHI, articulate key universal beliefs about the targeted population to justify a global response. A pamphlet I received during a visit to UNICEF's headquarters in New York City in 1997 helps to illustrate this. Titled "The Challenge to Nature," the opening section, which promotes the BFHI, states that it is only recently that "humans have tried to replace the natural means of feeding newborns which is given to every mammalian species on Earth" (UNICEF/WHO 1996, 7). The problem of the worldwide decline in breastfeeding is placed in the broadest of population parameters—that of all mammals. Humans, it tells us, comprise the only mammalian species that has challenged the natural order of things by replacing breast milk in the feeding of infants. The statement overlooks the fact that breastfeeding among humans (and some primates) is learned behavior for both mothers and infants (Jelliffe and Jelliffe 1978; Dettwyler 1987). There are indeed innate aspects of the process, but much trial and error is often necessary for successful breastfeeding by women.[9] If these statements are read as ways in which a political organization seeks to define a problem with regard to mothering and infant feeding, then it appears that humans (women) defy nature's intentions in rejecting the gift of their capacity to breastfeed. This logic situates the BFHI as a way to return humans (mothers) to their place in the naturalized hierarchy of the animal kingdom. It might seem that attention to a pamphlet's rhetoric is overthinking a public health program. However, in 2013 UNICEF's China office, in honor of World Breastfeeding Week, produced an animated video distributed to all UNICEF offices titled *Breastfeeding, Natural Love*, which depicts animals from pandas to whales breastfeeding their offspring.[10] The video's final sequences depict each young animal uttering the word *mama* as it gazes into its mother's eyes, except the human infant. Seated next to a can of infant formula with no mother in sight, the infant plaintively utters *mama*. We will see in later chapters how such representations of an essential, biological woman continue to undergird assumptions and practices in the implementation of the BFHI.

The pamphlet also targets culture and human ingenuity in the form of industrialization and modernization as culprits in the global decline in breastfeeding.

> The challenge to Nature took hold in the industrialized countries in the 20th century and especially after the Second World War, which had brought many more women into the workforce. Technological advances in packaged foods made it possible to offer breast milk substitutes to women trying to balance the pressures of their work both in and outside the home. . . . Hospitals tied to the rigorous schedules of industrialized societies encouraged the switch to regular bottle-feeding. "Baby's bottle" became a typical advertising image of modern "progress." (UNICEF/WHO 1996, 7)

This passage reveals a number of important cultural assumptions about mothering and infant feeding in relation to industrialization. Nature, as it is used in this passage, can be read not only as working in opposition to "culture" (industrialization and modernity) but also as a higher order. In this view, natural maternal nurturance through breastfeeding is thwarted by women's participation in the modernizing world (Scheper-Hughes 1987). These statements make it clear that good mothering and even infant survival are incompatible with women's participation in the work force and that children are best served when their mothers are relegated to the traditional spheres of home and family (Blum 1993, 302; Wolf 2010, 128). In a broader sense, the rhetorical strategies used in this pamphlet highlight an instance of the persistence and usefulness of the nature/culture opposition in defining gender at a time when new reproductive technologies appear to be diminishing these differences (Franklin, Lury and Stacey 2000, 7).

More practically, linking the loss of traditional lifeways and women's distance from nature in the BFHI pamphlets offers a rather simplistic interpretation of the reasons for the worldwide decline in breastfeeding. Such logic does not reflect the reality of most women's lives in either the past or the present. As our knowledge about breastfeeding gleaned from fine-grained ethnographic studies increases, researchers have shown that even women in "traditional" agrarian societies confront situations in which breastfeeding is incompatible with their work (Maher 1992; Levine 1988; Nerlove 1974). Levine suggests that the increasing use of breast milk substitutes in urban contexts reflects long-standing practices of supplementation when rural women's work is incompatible with the breastfeeding demands of infants. For example, she finds that in Nepal traditional supplementary foods are introduced early in infancy as a way to prepare infants to accept these foods at moments when women's agricultural work is incompatible with their additional responsibilities for childcare and breastfeeding (Levine 1988, 247). In making a case for breastfeeding and the BFHI, the pamphlet indirectly advocates a return to an ideal of the housewife and mother against which many women have fought in the interest of their social and economic autonomy (Wolf 2010). In a socialist nation such as China, which has promised women emancipation from the most oppressive aspects of patriarchy through employment in return for their support of national goals, this message is particularly poignant.

The language of the pamphlet also reflects a transition in public health policy and practice to what is called the new public health or health promotion. Established by the WHO's Ottawa Charter in 1986, the new public health directive emphasizes "an advocacy framework to enable communities and individuals to attain optimum health" (Awofeso 2004, 706).[11] As Peterson and Lupton show, this "is at its core a moral enterprise that involves prescriptions about how we should live our lives and conduct our bodies, both individually and collectively" (1997, 174). Health promotion emphasizes that individuals and populations are at risk of becoming ill in an ever more uncertain world. These risks can be found everywhere from the spatial and physical to the social and psychological realms (Peterson and Lupton 1997). The new public health also emphasizes the importance of an individual's participation in improving his or her health. Returning to the quote from the BFHI pamphlet examined earlier, we can see a similar argument advanced with regard to breastfeeding: environmental risks to infant health result from industrialization, women working outside the home, and technological advances in the mass production of infant formulas. These circumstances, the pamphlet suggests, have created a situation in which infants are at risk of death and disease because their mothers are not making the appropriately healthy choice to breastfeed. This argument illustrates how health promotion simultaneously identifies risky environments and behaviors that can create the possibility of one becoming ill and works on the assumption that individuals seek to maximize good health through self-management (Peterson 1997, 197). Caring for an infant adds a twist to this scenario, however, for a mother must balance not only the infant's immediate need to remain healthy but also the needs of her own well-being.

The response of UNICEF/WHO to the potential tension between a mother's needs and those of her infant is to focus on the child. The BFH, the pamphlet claims, will "put infants and children first . . . which will lead to the world's return to breastfeeding and put an end to thousands of infant deaths" (UNICEF/WHO 1996, 3). The solution proposed by UNICEF/WHO aims to set up hospitals and routines that promote rather than discourage breastfeeding. Women I met in the course of this study understood that they had become secondary players in the drama of creating new citizens. "They should make mother-friendly hospitals, since we are the ones who care for babies!" Wang Hong declared one day. Wang Hong and other women I met believed that *they* needed a supportive and nurturing environment so that they could be good mothers to their infants. But the stated goal of the BFHI and others like it is, first, to create an environment more conducive to breastfeeding by changing practices in urban hospitals and, second, to educate women about the benefits of breast milk for their infants.[12] Nowhere, except in the poster promoting health tonics described earlier, is the mother's well-being considered. Rather, the BFHI in its promotional materials and practices seems to assume that mothers need no help for themselves because their physiological characteristics will naturally see them through the process. At the same time, the policy urges mothers to subject themselves to institutionalized regulation and surveillance to help them become good mothers. This contradiction suggests the ways in which public health, in defining the possible risks to maternal and child health, conveys multiple layers of meanings and ideologies related to broader social and cultural dynamics. These rest on a logic that is articulated in the BFHI: the interests of individual mothers are relegated to larger institutional concerns with protecting future generations. Infant survival rather than maternal well-being in a program like the BFHI then becomes an international and national concern requiring that mothers be managed and monitored in the interests of maintaining a healthy nation and world.[13]

It should be clear from this brief discussion that the ideals of maternity and infant feeding espoused by these organizations are not neutral. Others have noted this tension. Van Esterik, writing on the issue, observed that breastfeeding also creates one of "the most difficult dilemmas in feminist thought and action—the sexual division of labor and the fit between women's productive and reproductive activities" (1989, 68). Breastfeeding, like pregnancy and birth, represents a contradiction between "the cultural and natural mother; that is, the socially constructed and the biological are inextricably intertwined" (Blum 1993, 291). On the one hand, women's biological ability to produce breast milk connects their bodies and behaviors to the realm of nature; the act can be seen as one that encourages "natural" maternal nurturance. On the other hand, infant feeding decisions and definitions of proper, adequate mothering can be viewed as culturally and temporally contingent (Scheper-Hughes 1987). The ambivalence about breastfeeding as a focus of study in feminist scholarship rests on the difficulty of reconciling the social and biological dimensions of mothering and is reflected in the relative dearth of research on it compared to topics like childbirth or new reproductive technologies.[14] Ultimately these tensions, whether we look at feminist scholarship or public health policy and practice that ties breastfeeding to biology—and its decline to modernization—create a myth of the "universal mother," who may then be targeted for intervention by public health agencies (Allen 2004).

Infant Feeding in Urban China

China presents a puzzling situation with regard to infant feeding. Pasternak and Wang (1985) found that despite supportive policies for breastfeeding, including workplace nurseries, extended paid maternity leaves, and minimal availability of commercial infant formula or other breast milk substitutes, fewer and fewer urban Chinese women were breastfeeding. They found that in 1950, 93 percent of urban women had breastfed their infants but by 1983 only 13 percent were doing so (435). Here was a country following all the recommended guidelines set by organizations like the WHO and UNICEF to support breastfeeding and a decline still occurred. The authors themselves could not explain their findings in light of the received wisdom about breastfeeding in developing countries and suggested that understanding decreases in breastfeeding rates in China required more complex frameworks of analysis (464). Although my project cannot directly respond to Pasternak and Wang's findings, they inspired me to focus on infant feeding practices and the interconnected spheres of motherhood, medicine, public health, and reproduction.

The following pages, then, seek to document that the process of becoming a mother in a baby-friendly Chinese hospital offers a window for viewing how global health policies, consumer culture, and national intervention in reproductive health operate on the ground. We learn how women navigate these forces as they make decisions about feeding their infants. Women's narratives about pregnancy, childbirth, and the early postpartum period in later chapters offer insights into questions about how individuals manage their lives in the face of powerful external influences. More specifically, a focus on becoming a mother in the context of a hospital gives us a ground-level view of how gender is constituted as both the projection and product of cultural and political symbols and discourses as well as the material experiences and pragmatic actions of individuals (Kaufert and Lock 1998). This work, then, builds on scholarship that has brought infant feeding as a part of reproduction to the center of social theory and has approached biomedicine as a symbolic system of beliefs that reproduces power relations, creates subject positions, and shapes embodied experiences.[15]

As originally conceived, this project sought to examine how becoming a mother offered insight into the ways in which Chinese women contended with the contradictory messages that arise from a deeply rooted tradition that celebrates Confucian notions of the "virtuous wife and good mother" (*xianqi liangmu*) and a socialist state that demanded that women participate actively in economic life as "capable women" (*nu qiang ren*).[16] However, the complex constellation of forces in 1990s Beijing, as I discovered throughout the course of my research, created expectations that charged women with far more than simply achieving a balance between traditional and socialist ideals of good mothers and capable women. In fact, when I began my research in Beijing in 1994, the term "capable woman" (*nu qiang ren*) denoted a woman who was too strong, too capable—who had, in fact, lost her femininity as she modeled herself along the lines of the socialist ideal. This transformation of a previously positive label into one that called attention to women's lack of feminine attributes is emblematic of changes in the construction of gender ideals in 1990s China.[17] In Beijing, books, magazines, and advertisements visually displayed these multiple messages. At a magazine stand, one could find cover photos in *Parenting* (*FuMu*), a Chinese-produced magazine, that featured well-groomed, smiling mothers with their children alongside books about women's psychology and others about the health and protection of pregnant mothers. Images of women as objects and subjects of consumption dominated the stand, which featured calendars with and posters of scantily dressed models—some of them western—embracing sleek cars or posing coyly for the camera as the main attraction.

I found conducting research amid this welter of mixed images and the rapidly changing environment of urban China daunting. Chance and the realities of conducting fieldwork in China determined my choice to work in a Beijing hospital. It was at this single site that I was able to observe and make some sense of the multiple forces that I was witnessing on a large scale throughout city at this particular moment in time. The hospital thus operated as a location where medicine, global economic and political forces, and gender ideals met the actions and interests of individual women as they made infant feeding decisions.

Populating a Research Project

The thirty women who form the heart of this study, through choice or insurance directives, received their prenatal care, gave birth to their children, and obtained postpartum treatment at the district level Number 35 Hospital in Beijing. Thirteen of these women had attained college, high school, or technical school educations and worked in white-collar jobs as administrators, nurses, or teachers. Eleven others, with either primary or middle school educations, were employed as factory workers or store clerks. What these twenty-four women shared was the status of their workplaces, for they all worked for state-owned institutions such as factories, schools, hospitals, or publishers.[18] These state-owned enterprises were among the last holdouts in China's move to a market economy and had a record of offering the most comprehensive benefits for women. A third group of six women were either small business owners or worked in a family business (*getihu*). These women's accounts broadened the scope of my findings because they worked closer to the margins of urban society and enjoyed less security than state workers.[19] As later chapters show, women's employment situations in the mid-1990s, in cities like Beijing, reflected broader changes occurring as a result of state-level policies to promote rapid industrialization; to decrease dependence on government financial support by enterprises in all sectors of the economy; and ultimately, to foster fast economic growth.

Beyond documenting how differences in employment and education in China affected women's reproductive lives, I used this sampling strategy to engage with the field of public health and policy making in a context within and beyond China. As discussed earlier, worldwide, researchers link rates of breastfeeding and the incidence of infant disease or malnutrition to maternal educational levels and types of maternal employment and promotion of commercial infant formula to new mothers.[20] While this strategy may be the only feasible way to address thorny issues on a global scale, it is precisely such an essentialist approach that promotes generalizations and stereotypes about mothers and overlooks local and individual beliefs, strategies, and practices (Allen 2004). One of the major contributions of my study, then, is that it adds concrete information about constraints and decisions made by a sample of women in urban China during a time of rapid change and suggests that a well-rounded understanding of infant feeding practices in any nation would benefit from more attention devoted to particular economic, social, and cultural configurations, as well as how such decisions relate to motherhood.[21]

With the hope of documenting the nature of women's daily lives at home and work as they became mothers, I initially sought permission to conduct field research in a few large work units or neighborhoods. Two factors made such a plan impossible. First, in 1994, because of heightened government scrutiny of foreign social science researchers, my hosts worried about finding units that would be willing to allow an anthropologist access to pregnant women. Second, because the one-child policy limited pregnancies, even the largest work units had so few pregnant women that I would need to work in an unwieldy number of locations. As an alternative, my thoughtful mentors at the Academy of Preventive Medicine helped arrange for me to conduct research at a local district-level hospital. At first I was concerned that being based in a hospital would limit my ability to understand women's daily lives as they became mothers. However, the drawbacks of working in a hospital setting quickly receded when I learned that the Number 35 Hospital had recently been awarded the status of a BFH by UNICEF/WHO. This development furnished an opportunity to better understand the daily realities of implementing a global public health initiative and how mothers, their family members, and health professionals made it work for them. The nurses and physicians who administered the "baby-friendly" program at the hospital and my observations and conversations with them—thus their voices—have a place in this book. The staff of the Obstetrics and Gynecology Department was comprised of all women, and many were mothers themselves. As they shepherded women through their pregnancies, births, and postpartum recoveries, they also guided me through the research process. Their insights, comments, personal stories, and observations advanced my own thinking about how women fared more generally in the post-Maoist reform era.

In addition to the formal connections to individuals I made through the Number 35 Hospital, my personal world was populated with a wide variety of friends, family, and serendipitous encounters with strangers. As so many researchers have discovered, taxi drivers are often their best informants regarding life on the ground in many countries (Melly 2017). Male taxi drivers, on discovering my research interests, would often fill the time during our travels with descriptions of the ways in which their wives negotiated motherhood, especially their struggles and triumphs with infant feeding, the early days of infancy, and returning to work after a maternity leave. Some drivers described their search for solutions and information on behalf of their wives in the early days after the birth of their child, the negotiations required between couples and their extended families about feeding and rearing an infant, and their own feelings about parenting and what futures their child would face in China. In addition to my frequent surprise about their willingness to chat with me about their personal lives, even in the context of an anonymous cab ride, these men's stories and insights often helped me formulate questions and ideas that I took back to the women I worked with at the Number 35 Hospital. Aside from these more anonymous contributions, friends made arrangements for me to visit other hospitals in Beijing to learn more about maternal and child health care. Through one friend, I was even allowed to visit a famous military hospital (usually not open to foreigners at all) where I met with physicians and nurses in the Obstetrics and Gynecology Department clinics and wards. These opportunities provided me with a broader sense of obstetric care in the city and served to help me understand the position of the Number 35 Hospital in this network of hospitals.

My courtship and eventual marriage to a Chinese man during my field research fundamentally shifted my relationships with women in the study group and the physicians, nurses, and other staff members at the hospital. Nurse Bai, with whom I worked on a daily basis in the obstetrics clinic, was the one who happily announced my marriage to all the women in the study, to her coworkers, and indeed to anyone who crossed the threshold of the clinic. She was particularly pleased that I was finally married. And she, like other women, perceived me as sharing certain common experiences. As one woman laughingly said to me on learning that I had recently married a Chinese man, "Now you know what it is like to have a Chinese mother-in-law!" A number of women who participated in this study became more frank with me on hearing of my marriage. Suddenly we were having discussions about sex lives, body and weight concerns, and relations with parents and in-laws, to name but a few. These discussions have helped to shape my understanding of women's lives within and outside the hospital as they became mothers despite the many differences between us.

Research visits with these women included numerous group discussions during hospital visits and breastfeeding classes, individual interviews at intervals during their pregnancies, births, and postpartum recoveries, and informal conversations at the hospital, in homes, or during shopping trips and meetings for tea, to name but a few. While uniformly interacting with all thirty women at regular intervals during the research, the nature of my relationship with each varied considerably. I formed closer, friendlier relationships with eight women in the group, who invited me to their homes, to restaurants for meals, or to sightsee at one of Beijing's many tourist locations. These women ranged from a seamstress with a middle school education who worked from her home to an editorial manager at a publishing house. Among all thirty, however, I was the first foreigner with whom they had spent extended periods of time. For thirteen women, I think the distance between us meant that I was able to establish only a formal rapport that was confined to the hospital. My relationships with ten other women existed somewhere between these two extremes. We would often meet at the Number 35 Hospital and then take a walk to the nearby department store café or hotel coffee shop to continue our conversations.

Material Matters: Advertising and Publishing about Motherhood and Infant Feeding

At times constant shifts in Beijing on many fronts made me wonder if I could ever grasp what all these changes meant or how they were being interpreted in terms of social values, norms, and ideals. Books, magazines, and advertisements helped anchor me at this time. For example, popular books about pregnancy, motherhood, and infant care had come to my attention during visits to China in 1991 and 1992. Browsing bookstores in Beijing and Harbin during these visits led to my discovery of dozens of titles devoted to these topics. As part of this study, over the course of my research, I purchased more than two hundred of these books from large urban bookstores in major shopping areas of Beijing, from local bookstores near the Number 35 Hospital and from local bookstands positioned at street corners throughout the city. Some of these advice manuals were also sold in the Number 35's lobby at its newly established bookstand alongside titles on such topics as health and aging, nutrition, and cooking. While this development may not seem startling to readers who are familiar with gift shops in hospitals where magazines and snacks are available, the bookstand represented a new use of hospital space for commercial purposes. Its presence signaled a response to changing policies that required hospitals to become financially independent of the government—selling books could make money. This change in policy for hospitals and the purchase and use of such books are discussed in some detail in later chapters. For now it is useful to point out that such cultural products, in their variety and volume and new locations, can reveal useful insights about some of the representations of motherhood, femininity, the female body, and babies that influenced women and how they fed their infants.

In addition to books, a diverse and widely available genre of popular magazines focused on family life, women, health, fashion, and home decorating was to be found at corner newsstands and bookstands throughout Beijing. While magazines had been available before the 1990s, the explosion of increasingly specialized ones was rather remarkable. For example, in 1992 and 1993, when I began to collect popular women's magazines in Beijing and Harbin, I discovered that there were only two or so titles consistently available at bookstores and corner stands. By 1995–96, however, I found it daunting to collect systematically magazines of this genre because there were so many available. These inexpensive magazines were published by Chinese entities and featured glossy, vibrant front and back covers enclosing pages of heavy newsprint-quality paper with articles, letters, cartoons, line drawnings, and blurry black and white photographs. Alongside these publications, in 1995 the Chinese-language version of *Vogue* magazine began to appear in bookstores and bookstands. Less remote than the thirteen or so McDonald's restaurants scattered throughout the city or the central shopping district at Wangfujing where stores like Benneton were establishing their presence, such magazine stands represented a material manifestation of the increasing presence of Euro-American popular culture in the local pedestrian and shopping spaces of Beijing. Differences in price, quality of paper, and artistic production notwithstanding, the availability of both types of magazines also help to situate the changing milieu in which women were becoming mothers, for they mark internal and external manifestations about the expectations and possibilities of this particular time in Beijing (Wu 2010, 152; Evans 1994, 2011).

Much as these forms of print media served to offer some concrete sense of ideals and desires surrounding motherhood and reproduction, advertisements produced by the Chinese government and commercial entities provided yet another material means with which to understand these manifestations. These promotions were not aimed simply at a select group of educated citizens as I realized during my daily commute to the hospital. Bicycling to the subway station, for example, I regularly passed a colorful painted billboard depicting a smiling couple holding hands with their single child, surrounded by rockets, a computer, and a chemistry beaker; underneath in bright red characters it exhorted viewers, "Develop the Nation." At the subway platform, one day I found myself in front of the Gerber baby foods baby! In a series of glossy, backlit advertisements placed directly across from the subway platform where, the day before, these posters had promoted a Chinese brand of washing machines and air conditioners, Gerber baby foods were being marketed to subway riders. Inspired by this startling change on my daily commute, I intermittently photographed and collected advertisements of foreign and Chinese goods related to mothers and children. These materials served to mark the way these commodities were making their way into the daily visual and material worlds of ordinary Chinese people. But later a taxi driver reminded me that such posters and billboards do not inhibit the Chinese government's use of these media as a way to promote its official agenda. So I also sporadically collected images of government-sponsored posters and billboards related to reproduction. While these media are not a primary focus of this book, their presence serves as a reminder that reproduction remains central to the balance between state control and a market economy that characterized 1990s China and continues to the present day.

Ultimately, the systematic aspects of the research process, such as the creation of sample groups representing different types of employment available to women, collecting popular books and magazines, and documenting the routines of the obstetrics clinic and wards in the Number 35 Hospital, were meant to address questions about how to more thoroughly understand women's decisions and practices as they became mothers in relation to global and national public health concerns and policies. At the same time, the constantly changing physical, cultural, social, and economic milieu that characterized Beijing offered reminders and insights into the fundamental instability inherent in attempting to document people's lives. These realities required making choices about how best to represent what I learned. Throughout much of the book, I have chosen to present an array of voices, observations, and insights from among the thirty women in the research sample rather than focusing on a few individuals in more depth as they navigated pregnancy, childbirth, and motherhood. This decision arose from my desire to highlight the similarities and differences in the ways that women become mothers rather than the experiences of a few key respondents.[22] The drawback to this decision is that readers may not feel that they have come to know anyone in this book and the women's individuality may seem lost. Yet, in the interest of responding to the homogenization of women's reproductive lives in relation to global and state policies and agendas, I believe it is most useful to highlight how women with different life histories, circumstances, interests, and desires found multiple routes to successfully feeding their infants.

Infant Feeding and Social Theory

In a 2011 editorial in the *International Breastfeeding Journal*, Lisa Amir suggested that public health researchers must incorporate not only qualitative methods but also the social theories of Bourdieu and others to better understand infant feeding practices and health behavior more generally (2011). The call to situate infant feeding decisions and practices in social theory offers a new response from public health professionals to the continuing, challenging efforts to understand these decisions using the tools of survey data (Amir 2011). The prospect of how best to use theory in developing our understanding of infant feeding in this book requires considering a complex array of actors and institutions—from mothers and infants, husbands, families, health care professionals, hospitals, and state policies and programs to global public health initiatives. Given the number of interests, experiences, and actions that arise in this constellation, it seems best to avoid identifying an overarching theoretical frame through which we might better understand women and their infant feeding decisions and practices. To this end, I draw on a variety of theories throughout the book that help to illuminate the particular circumstances at hand.

To create at least a heuristic model of the possibilities, pragmatics, and practices that women negotiate as they become mothers and make infant feeding decisions, I draw on the idea of social navigation (Tsing 2010). In Anna Tsing's view, the term *navigation* conveys the way individuals, at times, actively plot and steer themselves through particular moments and in others simply go with the flow and follow the path that arises before them. Navigation thus encapsulates theoretical approaches that seek to understand when and how ordinary people exert their agency in the face of multiple, changeable circumstances (420). In this way, we can tease out the nature of the institutional and internalized technologies of the self, developed by Foucault, and the actions, aspirations, and pragmatics of individuals (Bourdieu 1977; de Certeau 1988; Foucault 1987). In finding ways to understand the terrain to be navigated around infant feeding in 1990s China, one of the key theoretical frames that arises throughout the book draws on Foucault's concepts of modern power and governance (or, in shorthand, biopolitics). As Susan Greenhalgh shows in her work on China's population policy, "To a growing extent modern power is power over life, in the biological sense, and modern governance is the governance of human life—that is the administration and cultivation of individual and collective life, health, and welfare" (2010, 12).

I have learned through this project that, while the women I worked with dealt with seemingly similar circumstances and their strategies reflect responses to the biopolitics of infant feeding and the one-child policy, they acted according to what made sense given their individual circumstances, social relations, and subjectivities. I focus, then, on the dynamics of everyday agency among these women as they navigated within the boundaries created by mid-1990s Chinese society. Lyn Parker and Laura Dales reinforce this approach by suggesting that there is much to gain by looking at agency "as relational empowerment, cultural practice or capability [which] allows us to consider meaning of a variety of micro-level practices, beliefs, and interpersonal engagements" (2015, 167). Following in the footsteps of feminist scholars of Asia and beyond, this book thus aims to situate the dynamics of power and agency in ways that explore what this means in women's lives without losing sight of the limitations of such a focus.[23] To this end I use the notion of creative pragmatism to capture women's individual responses to both immediate and distant constraints and possibilities as they carried and then cared for their only child (Lock and Kaufert 1998; Mohanty 1991). Creative pragmatism both encapsulates the uniqueness of individual responses to particular situations and acknowledges the limitations that shape these responses. When a woman, for instance, leaves a mandatory breastfeeding class early because she finds it irrelevant to her situation, or when a nurse bends the rules of a global health policy to help a patient, we may see how such actions both highlight the constraints these women must work within and the individual nature of their responses.[24]

Much as the metaphor of navigation conveys possibilities for maneuvering or going with the flow, it also assumes the existence of unforeseen and particular obstacles, as well as helpful structures. Moving beyond the literal metaphor, we know that external forces do not necessarily have to be structural but can also be symbolic or representational in nature and indeed often operate at both levels simultaneously. So, for example, China's one-child policy may be viewed as a structural response to the political and economic problem of overpopulation. Yet the policy and its goals also represent aspirations of modernity and prosperity for the nation. In light of these agendas, it becomes possible to understand that women might respond to the one-child policy as a personal experience, a political reality, and a national and personal aspiration simultaneously and may place different emphases on these dimensions of the policy in their own lives.[25]

Finally, we must attend to the fact that bearing and feeding an infant, whether by breast or bottle, highlight the ways in which women navigate their own bodies and those of their infants. Throughout the book I draw on different theories of the body that can situate these women's lives in broader discussions and findings about infant feeding and reproduction. Theories about the body attune us to the ways in which mothers and infants are simultaneously individually experienced, material bodies, symbolic bodies, and social and political bodies subject to constraints and regulation (Scheper-Hughes and Lock 1987). For example, when looking at global and national policies aimed at increasing breastfeeding, Foucault's notion of biopower helps clarify how states and organizations like the WHO established that infant feeding practices require regulation through policies and laws. At the same time the workings of biopower became visible through the regulation of bodies as women in this study participated in the BFHI (Foucault 2007 in Greenhalgh 2010).

To attend to the individual, materially experienced bodies of the women in this book, I draw on feminist and anthropological scholarship that seeks to bring the embodied work and experiences of infant feeding and reproduction to our attention (Stearns 2013; Shaw and Bartlett 2010). Until recently, feminist scholars have primarily analyzed the ideological and cultural aspects of breastfeeding and largely avoided the bodily aspects of the process (Stearns 2013). Indeed, pregnancy, childbirth, and breastfeeding represent a conundrum in feminist theory. The universal biological processes of reproduction potentially anchor women in a maternal identity to the exclusion of other identities. These may serve as justification for or reinforce gender hierarchies, and may obscure our understanding of differences among women (Hird 2007, 3). Anthropologist Elly Teman's study of pregnancy and surrogacy makes clear that pregnancy itself does not "naturally" transform women into mothers. She suggests that "we view pregnancy as an organic, biological process, but also a bodily site upon which identity work is taken" (2010, 50). Infant feeding—whether breastfeeding or not—may represent another time when women may "discursively and bodily construct a particular self-identity and role" (50). In broader theoretical terms, infant feeding provides an opportunity to understand, as Turner suggests, that the body is "both subjective and objective, meaningful and material, personal and social, and can be considered the 'material infrastructure' of the productions of selves, belongings and identities" (Turner 1994, quoted in Van Walputte 2004, 256). Framing the process of becoming a mother and nourishing an infant in terms of navigation thus helps to bring out the ways in which the specific domains of reproduction, public health, and biomedicine are made up of knowledge and beliefs that replicate power relations, create possible identities for individuals, and shape their embodied experience.[26]

The particular forms that constrain, as well as create, possibilities for women become clear in the hospital setting.[27] The space of a hospital can represent the government's desire for healthy, productive future citizens. Hospital workers seek to ensure, with limited resources, that healthy mothers and infants leave their clinics and wards. Companies look for new customers to whom to promote their products, while women search for solutions to the bodily, social, and personal changes wrought by motherhood. But women also operate in other contexts, such as family and work, where they must manage the expectations of family members and employers. Most often their families included their mothers and mothers-in-law, and generally these older women adhered to time-honored routines around pregnancy, childbirth, and infant feeding that conflicted with the signals emanating from the media and "modern" experts.[28] Women's worries about how to manage their femininity and relations with their husbands also reflected the increasing importance in urban China of conjugal relationships. At work women sought to balance their pregnant and lactating bodies with the demands of their jobs. In sum my use of navigation theoretically and conceptually grounds a complex time for women as they became mothers without losing sight of both the constraints and possibilities that ordered their lives.

While navigation provides a frame for tracing the paths that these women took, I also draw on the idea of potentiality to highlight how infant feeding embodies a future for the state, the family, and the child (Zhu 2013). As Taussig, Hoeyer, and Helmreich (2013) show us, potentiality projects into the future, but, unlike expectations or promises, "It makes a moral claim on others to act" (S10). Breastfeeding certainly makes a moral claim on all mothers. The logic of potentiality in the realm of infant feeding resides in the beliefs that breast milk can minimize infant disease and death and maximize the health and intelligence of future citizens. Mothers, then, have within their very bodies the means to ensure the future of their children and the nation. Breastfeeding thus becomes a moral obligation. Good mothers breastfeed, and bad mothers do not.

Potentiality also captures these dynamics as they occur in other contexts. For example, the shift in public health to an emphasis on health promotion, discussed above, frames individual and community well-being as something at risk in an increasingly unreliable world. The public's health relies on the moral obligation of individuals to do all that they can to maximize their health. This kind of reasoning helps to justify the global institutional efforts made by organizations like the WHO and UNICEF to induce mothers to breastfeed their infants. Within the family, new mothers encounter the potentiality in their recoveries from childbirth. New mothers discover that to ensure their long-term health they must adhere to postpartum traditions that go against their modern sensibilities. If they do not adhere to such customs, these women could face chronic illnesses as they get older. Throughout the book, then, I draw on the different scales and temporal nature of potentiality to highlight the ways in which the possibilities of an uncertain future, whether individual, familial, national, or global, come to be expressed in infant feeding practices. In sum navigation and potentiality work as broad webs within which the relevant and appropriate theoretical frames may be used throughout the book.

Conceptions: 1990s China and Maternal Governance

Some readers may wonder: why read about infant feeding in 1990s China? Our curiosity about understanding China in the present day perhaps stems from the fact that the country seems to be changing at lightning speed and in grand, monumental ways. We want to better understand what is happening now, how it is happening, and what these changes might mean for China, the world, and at times our own lives. I empathize with these desires.

The mid-1990s were marked by several crucial political, social, and economic changes that spurred China into the twenty-first century. These changes occurred at different speeds and different levels of society. Some of the changes most relevant to this book range from the state's adoption and design of global policies and practices for reproductive and child health to shifts in the one-child policy, the introduction of urban homeownership, an explosion of foreign and domestic consumer goods, institution of a five-day work week, and increasingly market-driven employment practices. By focusing on a group of women in the mid-1990s from their pregnancies and recoveries from childbirth through their decisions about feeding their infants, we can learn through their eyes how such changes were navigated. To satisfy our questions and curiosity about contemporary China, and to create a longer analytical lens connecting the recent past to the present, I bring developments about infant feeding in the twenty-first century to our attention throughout the book.

It was hard to miss some of the more obvious changes in Beijing from the time of my first visit in 1985, when the economic reforms began to have a material impact, to the time of my primary field research in 1994–96, when China was seeking more connections with outside entities, including the WHO and the World Trade Organization. Most superficially, the city was under construction. Tall, shiny, glass-sided hotels and office buildings were replacing the concrete and brick buildings of the 1950s. No longer were shoppers limited to dank, poorly lit neighborhood stores carrying mostly Chinese goods. Women could now choose to buy foreign-produced infant formula in brightly lit, air-conditioned department stores with expansive displays and counters of imported and domestic cosmetics, housewares, jewelry, food, and clothing. The availability of such consumer goods extended to the small family-owned shops found in most neighborhoods, where people could purchase Nestle's ice cream and Dove chocolate bars, Fuji film, Tide laundry detergent, and Coca-Cola alongside daily necessities such as Chinese-produced toilet paper, batteries, beer, and laundry soap. Moreover, staple foods like rice, wheat flour, sugar, and cooking oil were no longer rationed, resulting in an expanded variety of baked goods and convenience foods available at local shops and the establishment of numerous small restaurants.

Most scholars of China associate the changes that began in the 1990s with Deng Xiaoping's 1992 Southern Tour during which he put forth an agenda to further deepen economic reforms and open doors to trade with the world (Zhao 1993). China's foreign trade increased from US$21 billion in 1978 to more than $300 billion in 1997 and more than $1.15 trillion in 2004. Closed under the Chinese Communist Party (CCP) in 1949, the Shanghai Stock Market reopened in 1990, reflecting a state-level commitment to bringing more capitalist institutions to China's economic scene.[29] State-owned enterprises, the anchors of China's centrally planned economy since the 1950s, accelerated their transformations into either "modern corporations" or failing legacies of central planning (Putterman and Dong 2002). China's integration into the global economy accelerated after 1992 as well: its share of the world's export market expanded from 1.6 percent in 1985 to 4.8 percent in 1995. By 1994 China was the largest recipient of foreign direct investment, second only to the United States. Entry into the World Trade Organization in 2001 established China's key role in global trade and commerce. The macrolevel economic changes percolated through to individuals and households as well. While incomes rose rapidly from 1985 to the time of my research in 1994, looking at urban households' possession of major durable consumer goods between these years provides a sense of the material changes occurring in people's lives. For example, ownership of refrigerators increased from 6.58 per 100 households in 1985 to 56.68 in 1993; color televisions owned by 17.21 per 100 households in 1985 increased to 79.46 in 1993; and washing machines owned by 48.29 per 100 households in 1985 increased to 86.38 in 1993 according to the *Statistical Yearbook of China* (China Statistical Bureau 1994, 262). When my research began in late 1994, the effects of the shifts in policy after Deng's tour were already appearing in daily life. The women of this book show us what life was like at this turning point before China's extensive economic stratification and emergent middle class in the twenty-first century.

It is important to note that, while many of these transformations touched larger urban areas, most of the population, concentrated in the countryside, did not benefit equally from globalization and market socialism—a problem that other scholars have addressed (Solinger 1995; Jacka 2006; Rofel 1999, 2007). Nor should anyone assume that all citizens experienced the transformations that marked cities like Beijing in similar ways. Access to previously scarce Chinese goods and a variety of foreign commodities in the everyday lives of the women whose stories form the heart of this book represents more than a change in the material conditions of life resulting from shifts in state policy and the introduction of limited forms of capitalism in China. As we learn in chapter 4, for example, some mothers' concerns about losing weight after pregnancy reveal that social and cultural values taking hold under these new material conditions were influencing ideas about femininity and the female body that differed from the "iron girl" ideal of earlier socialist periods.[30]

China's efforts to modernize and develop its economy meant that in the workplace, women could take advantage of the newly instituted five-day work week, which created more opportunities for leisure activities such as shopping, bowling, dancing, learning English, and weekend travel. People were thinking in new ways about how to live and make a living. The phrase in the air in mid-1990s Beijing was *xiahai* (jump into the sea), which referred to those who sought to leave their secure but low-paying state jobs for positions in the riskier, newly developing private sector. This meant that some found employment in the increasing numbers of joint-venture companies formed between Chinese and foreign firms. Entrepreneurial individuals began to establish small businesses, from tailor shops and beauty salons to real estate offices and computer consulting companies.

Yet the job security, maternity leaves, child care facilities, and employment opportunities that had been a hallmark of the socialist agenda to liberate women during the Maoist years and the early years of reform started slipping away. As state and private enterprises sought ways to cut costs and increase efficiency in a competitive economic environment, catering to women's reproductive issues was deemed too costly. Maternity leaves, maternity insurance, and the belief that women's loyalties were divided between work and home helped justify measures that in the end excluded many women from the workplace.[31] And so at the very time when new possibilities for redefining participation in China's economic growth were appearing, many women were anxious about the stability of their work situation, and older women remembered with nostalgia the socialist programs that had protected vulnerable members of society (Honig and Hershatter 1988; Evans 1994; Rofel 1999).

In this ever-shifting milieu, managing a home and rearing a child began to represent an acceptable, and for some women desirable, alternative to full-time employment. Life without outside work for some seemed logical in light of the emphasis on family nutrition, childhood development, and time management promoted in the new, glossy women's magazines found at bookstands throughout the city. Advertising in these publications conveyed the idea that women's responsibilities for the family required more than good management skills but also an ability to consume wisely.[32] Changing policies in the mid-1990s that allowed city residents to purchase apartments reinforced the importance of home and the family. In 2012 the homeownership rate reached 85 percent (Gan 2013; Goodman 2014; Tomba 2009). As a result, the physical spaces of the home reflected trends in domesticity and consumption. Redecorating an apartment by covering concrete floors with parquet wood, installing crown molding and wallpaper over white plaster walls, and furnishing living rooms with leather sofas and large television sets had become not only permissible but desirable among many urbanites (Davis 2000; Zhang 2010). Homeownership or aspirations to own a home in the city also raised questions about how extended families might live together or not. Beepers made by foreign companies such as Motorola and Siemens provided an inexpensive means of communication for the many Beijing residents who were on years-long waiting lists for home phone installation. Industrious individual efforts to accumulate wealth and consume rather than participating in a system of state-managed production and consumption meant that many citizens no longer found it necessary to conform to many older socialist government ideals. Moreover, the lure of more than a billion customers brought many foreign companies to China, eager to sell their products and the accoutrements of a more cosmopolitan lifestyle.[33] Surfacing in the 1990s, these material changes underlie the emergence of a middle class in the twenty-first century and changes in feminine subjectivity and family relationships.[34]

Maternal Governance

These dazzling changes have prompted outside observers to argue that state intervention in the more mundane aspects of citizens' lives was fading.[35] However, much as it appeared that the state had retreated in many aspects of Chinese people's lives at this time, reproduction remained a realm where government interests and agendas were still clearly present and, with the BFHI, expanding.[36] For many readers, the one-child policy represents the Chinese government's most draconian interference in individual human rights. The early 1990s, for the state, represented an important turning point in China's population growth. Susan Greenhalgh shows how planners and policy makers saw this time period as one requiring vigilance in enforcing the policy as the number of women in their childbearing years reached a critical mass (Greenhalgh 2010, 41). Without strict adherence, it was anticipated that China's population growth would outstrip the country's economic gains. But by the mid-1990s, as fertility levels dropped below replacement levels and market socialism accelerated, the quality of China's newest citizens became a focus of both the state and families (58). While always a part of the birth-planning equation, the urgency of reducing the size of the population overshadowed concerns about how to produce individuals whose decisions would advance China's modernization project (41).[37] The women in this study thus straddled a crucial moment in the implementation of the one-child policy where adherence to the policy itself no longer sufficed. It was equally important to raise a physically and mentally superior citizen to see China on to its rightful place in the global power structure.

The Chinese government justified its attempt to control household decisions on grounds similar to those used to promote the BFHI; these policies would bring about economic development and thus raise the standard of living of its citizens.[38] Furthermore, China's adoption of other multilateral health policies aimed at reducing maternal mortality rates, guaranteeing maternity care, and preventing infant formula companies from promoting their products in hospitals at once institutionalized global standards of health practices and reinforced the legitimacy of government interest in reproduction. China's acceptance of these international standards for maternal and child health care also represents an important instance outside the economic domain in which Chinese officialdom embraced foreign practices and values.[39] Reproduction, then, becomes a lens through which the agendas and assumptions that constitute market socialism and multilateral health policies are rendered more visible. In doing so, we can see the beginnings in the 1990s of what Greenhalgh argues is a transition from a state-centered form of governance to governance by a variety of entities, such as the WHO or UNICEF or even infant formula companies, which bring different values and ideals to the task of "managing and perfecting China's society" (2010, 41). Among the women in this study, we also see that China's infant feeding policies and programs facilitate "more purely self-interested, self-governing reproductive subjects" (41).

I use the term *maternal governance* throughout the book as a shorthand term to encapsulate the expansion of the forms of governance in women's lives in the mid-1990s. The microdetails of women's decisions refract the broader social changes described above through state and global health policy agendas, consumer culture, and the emergence of new possibilities of self-governance at this crucial moment for both China and individual women. By documenting these shifts throughout the book, we can see how many laid the groundwork for practices and ideas about mothering and infant feeding in twenty-first-century China.

To most effectively explore these policies and changes and the ways in which mothers navigated them as they made decisions about caring for their infants, I have structured the book so that Chapter 1, "From Global to Local: Situating Motherhood and Infant Feeding," looks at how motherhood, reproduction, infant feeding, an emerging consumer culture, and new feminine bodily ideals took shape in 1990s China. The chapter also documents a contradiction inherent in global and Chinese breastfeeding policies: mothers are naturally suited to nurturing children, but to be successful, mothers require the assistance, regulation, and surveillance of national and international programs like the BFHI and institutions like the WHO.

Chapter 2, "Nature and Science: Making Modern Mothers in the Baby-Friendly Hospital," takes us to the Number 35 Hospital's obstetrics clinic. Looking at the spaces of the obstetrics clinic, observing breastfeeding classes, and following discussions with pregnant women, this chapter makes clear that the BFH seeks to encourage breastfeeding by representing the practice as natural, scientific, and ultimately modern. However, consumer products and their advertisements also began to appear in the hospital at this time, and women encountered posters of sexualized images of mothers and infants promoting maternal health tonics. We learn about the multiple responses adopted by women as they confronted these mixed messages about how best to mother their infants. This chapter's attention to the discursive and spatial dynamics designed to encourage women to breastfeed builds on recent feminist scholarly critiques of the contradictions found in breastfeeding programs like the BFHI as natural and yet requiring expert assistance (Liamputtong 2007; Dykes and Hall-Moran 2009). The appearance of popular media in hospital spaces just as my research began also captures a crucial turning point when new agents of maternal governance arrived in the public domain.

Chapter 3, "Anticipating Motherhood," takes up ways of knowing about pregnancy and infant feeding among the women in this study. We see that women did not actively seek to learn about their pregnancies from the hundreds of popular books available for purchase in the hospital, at bookstores, and at local newsstands. Instead, these women relied on the nurses and doctors to oversee and anticipate their medical needs and on their older female kin and friends to meet their nonmedical needs. Women's reliance on the expert knowledge of professionals and their experienced mothers rather than advice books provides insight into how women went about learning how to be good mothers. Moreover, we see their reactions to the material manifestations of new state-directed pressures to produce a high-quality child-citizen. In addition to developing an understanding of how women approached their pregnancies, the chapter provides an analysis of a sample of the popular pregnancy books for sale in the hospital lobby. These books portend a new family configuration for the care of pregnant women in which husbands replace mothers and mothers-in-law. Tracing the promotion of ideals of conjugal intimacy and documenting women's responses to them, this study expands our understanding of the workings of what Yan sees as the rise in individualization in China shaped by the state (2009).

Readers will no doubt notice that there is no chapter on childbirth in this book. While there is much to say about childbirth in China in the 1990s and the twenty-first century, in the context of the BFH, childbirth itself is not a crucial component of the initiative. Moreover, in the 1990s, pregnant women, hospital staff, and female kin did not view childbirth as a definitive moment in becoming a mother. I have thus chosen not to include childbirth in the book.

Chapter 4, "Between Hospital and Home: Childbirth, Infant Feeding, and 'Sitting the Month,'" explores how new mothers navigate between traditional postpartum practices overseen by their mothers or mothers-in-law, which are designed to strengthen their bodies, and modern pressures to recover their prepregnancy bodily shape.

In doing so, these new mothers draw on notions of tradition, science, nature, and modernity to develop a path to recovery for themselves and to make decisions about how best to nurture their infants. Women's return to the workplace brought infant feeding and child care into focus as they made decisions with potential long-term consequences. Chapter 5, "Maternal Maneuvers: Between Home and Work," shows the variety of ways in which women balance their desire for a healthy and intelligent child with their work lives, marital relationships, and sense of self. We learn that women's decisions about whether or not to breastfeed formed part of a pragmatic calculus in anticipation of their own, and their child's, future. Together these chapters extend our understanding of the complexities of infant feeding in a rapidly changing society. Finally, as mothers recover from childbirth and return to work, we see the unfolding of the earliest decisions Chinese women make as mothers: how best to nourish them. Much as Teresa Kuan found in her recent study of middle-class mothers in China, these new mothers did not simply internalize and accept state agendas to improve China's population quality or global health policies (Kuan 2015).

Audiences

My hope is that a long-term ethnographic study of Chinese women as they become mothers and make decisions about how to feed their infants will engage readers in a number of fields. For those with an interest in infant feeding from a public health perspective, this book provides the fine-grained, long-term ethnographic information essential to understanding the ways in which mothers make infant feeding decisions. It also complements the larger-scale, shorter-term research on infant feeding that helps us to see national or global patterns of breast and bottle feeding. This book expands our lens beyond factors that facilitate or inhibit breastfeeding to consider the contexts—cultural, political, economic, and social—that shape women's ideas about and experiences with mothering and infant feeding.[40] Those with an interest in what the implementation of a global health policy looks like on the ground will find that the exigencies of local circumstances, individual interests, and histories, and national agendas and interests shape universal, institutionalized efforts to bring about changes in health behavior in unanticipated ways both in implementing policy and in individuals' responses. Anthropologists interested in reproduction and infant feeding will find a case study that helps to situate breastfeeding as an embodied practice and a biocultural phenomenon shaped by economic, political, and social dynamics. As the first long-term ethnographic study of infant feeding and the BFHI in China, readers with an interest in China should find that this book extends our understanding of the effects of the one-child policy in women's lives and provides a context for contemporary research on mothering and parenting more generally. It also makes visible the crucial shifts in maternal governance from state policy and family dynamics to the increasing importance of self-governance through expansions of new agents, including global health organizations and China's emerging consumer culture. Beyond these audiences, I hope this book reaches those seeking to better understand the lives of Chinese women and their experiences with pregnancy, postpartum recovery, and infant feeding amid the rapid economic and social changes of post-reform China.

CHAPTER ONE

From Global to Local

Situating Motherhood and Infant Feeding

Introduction

As they prepared to give birth in a BFH, where exclusive breastfeeding for at least six months was promoted, women at the Number 35 Hospital were preoccupied with questions about how best to nourish their infants. For example, Zhai Xiurong, a twenty-five-year-old factory manager in her fifth month of pregnancy, talked about the importance of raising her only child to participate successfully in a more modern China—by feeding him foreign-produced infant formula.

> China is developing quickly and becoming more modern; I want my child to benefit from these advances. The traditional ways are not good. . . . The foreign brand of infant formula is expensive, but I don't believe that the Chinese formula companies are reliable. Who controls them? The foreign companies have international standards that they have developed, and they are more scientific. So I feel foreign products are safer and have better nutrition. Some of them even have more nutrients than breast milk!

Science, safety, and nutrition, for Zhai Xiurong, come packaged in more expensive foreign-produced infant formula. Literally, consuming this product serves in her mind as a way to help realize her child's potential to become a citizen of a modern, cosmopolitan China. From our vantage point in 2017, Xiurong's observations seem prescient. China's 2008 scandal involving Chinese-made infant formula tainted with melamime caused eight infant deaths and sickened thousands of babies[1] (*New York Times*, September 22, 2008). Incidents involving tainted formula continue to occur in China and other countries, including the United States. The safety and quality of infant formula are taken up in later chapters where women consider their options for feeding their newborns.

As she expressed concern about balancing the needs of her child and her desire for a slim body, Cui Zhuhong, a twenty-seven-year-old office worker two months postpartum explained, "I think that if a baby is healthy and has been breastfed during the first months after birth, it is alright to give it formula. . . . Breastfeeding makes it difficult to lose weight. I just felt too fat, and I knew I couldn't diet while breastfeeding, so after six weeks I stopped." As Zhuhong's statement indicates, despite hearing the strong message that breastfeeding provides better nourishment than the bottle, she—and others, as we shall learn—found herself balancing her needs with those of her infant, not convinced that breastfeeding was best for her or her child. Wu Qiuping, a twenty-five-year-old factory worker in her eighth month, however, stated that she believed breastfeeding was the way to ensure her child's healthy development: "Breastfeeding is the way to provide the best nutrition for my child. I want to raise a strong, healthy, and intelligent child, and since coming to the Number 35 Hospital I have learned that breast milk provides all the nutrition it will need." Qiuping's comments indicate that some women found the BFHI message "breast is best" convincing. These narratives reflect the potentials and pragmatics that women balanced when making decisions about how to feed their infants. They also help remind us that infant feeding decisions are more than an extension of biological reproduction but reside firmly as a part of social reproduction. Writing about the politics of breastfeeding, comparative literature scholar Jules Law makes clear the distinction: "Lactation is a reproductive phenomenon that takes place in a woman's body; infant feeding is a social activity in which the bodies, prerogatives, obligations of multiple citizens converge" (2000, 442).

This chapter outlines the contours of the historical, political, and economic landscape surrounding infant feeding that give shape and definition to the ways women, their families, and health professionals navigated infant feeding and policy decisions in the Number 35 Hospital. The first section looks at the relationship between public health and the problematizing of infant feeding to tease out some key assumptions that shape policies like that of the BFHI. Turning to the Chinese state, the chapter explores how adoption of a global health policy like the BFHI at once intersects and serves broader national interests centered on population quality, citizenship, and the future.[2] Moving beyond the realm of policy and politics, the chapter provides an overview of the consumer culture developing in 1990s China that brought about material and symbolic shifts in ideals of motherhood and femininity. These changes embodied new and old potentials about how to be a mother, wife, and worker in urban China.

"Breast Is Best": Infant Feeding as a Public Health Problem

> Breastfeeding is the cheapest, most effective life saver in history.
> (UNICEF press release, 2013)

Infant feeding as a focus of public health research and intervention dates back to the late nineteenth century. A brief sketch of this history here situates more contemporary concerns about infant feeding and motherhood as central to global and public health. In the United States in the early twentieth century, for example, infant feeding and mothering operated as a repository for anxieties about nation building, population quality, immigration, race, and class (Blum 1999, 182–83).[3] At stake was the creation of a strong, healthy population for the nation. Infant survival and health thus became public problems to be solved. Studies have shown how responses to these anxieties resulted in the development of public health programs that targeted mothers who did not measure up, namely, those women who were not white and middle class.[4] Framed in terms of the ideals of middle-class white women, policies and programs aimed at improving infant mortality rates called for good mothering, defined as staying home full time and breastfeeding (23). However, by the mid-twentieth century, with the availability of mass-produced infant formulas, bottle-feeding came to be associated with science and modernity.[5] This shift maintained the critical division between who could be a good mother and who could not, but it reversed the criteria so that women who could afford infant formula represented the ideal, forward-looking, modern, and scientifically oriented mother. Backward traditional mothers were the ones to resort to breastfeeding. The switches between breast- and bottle-feeding as more scientific exemplify how infant feeding is situated in the realm of social imperatives rather than biological reproduction over time and place.

The role of medical expertise and the commercial development of infant formula beginning in the early twentieth century also informs public health's current interest in managing infant feeding. Physicians during the twentieth century in the United States, according to historian Rima Apple (1987), staked a claim to infant health and nutrition for reasons of self-interest and humanitarianism.[6] The creation of the role of the medical expert, and in particular pediatrics as a medical specialty, beginning in the 1930s occurred in tandem with increasing availability of commercial infant formulas. Apple's research shows that over time these developments brought about the ideal of "scientific motherhood."[7] The "scientific" mother relied on the advice of medical experts and scientifically produced infant formulas to raise a modern child.

These developments, if we fast-forward to the 1970s, led to a reliance on medical expertise and science to help solve a crisis in developing countries, where the use of infant formula was associated with increasing numbers of infant deaths. Some readers may remember the boycott against Nestle, starting in the 1970s, in response to the widespread and deceptive marketing of its infant formula to mothers in less economically developed countries. Nestle was accused of offering free infant formula samples to women in hospitals, knowing that most could not afford to purchase the formula once they returned home. The company was also faulted for distributing infant formula in packaging without instructions in the local language so that reconstituting the powder might lead to errors and ultimately would compromise the health of infants. Bribing hospital officials, impersonating nurses on maternity wards in order to distribute formula samples, and contributing infant formula to humanitarian aid efforts were all charges leveled at Nestle. More generally, researchers have sought and continue to seek the key factors that determine whether women breastfeed or use infant formula and to explain worldwide declines in breastfeeding since the 1950s.[8]

Most approaches to explaining declines in breastfeeding assume that there exist potentially universal or ubiquitous forces that shape individual behavior. Thus, large-scale surveys continue to seek to document the myriad determinants of infant feeding.[9] From educational background, ethnic origin, and employment to urban or rural residence, number of children, and age, key correlations among such variables are sought to explain women's infant feeding practices and in particular their decisions to use infant formula. Correlations in such surveys between maternal education levels or types of employment and breastfeeding suggest that women with more education tend to breastfeed their children, while those who must work in the labor force do not breastfeed or do so for only a few weeks.[10] These findings have led researchers and policy makers to home in on the lives of less-educated, urban, wage-earning women who are not as likely to breastfeed. In essence, public health practitioners and policy makers use scientific methods to identify universal determinants that encourage or discourage breastfeeding. These factors inform the design of better programs aimed at changing individual behavior, and saving infants from death and disease in the global south.[11] Importantly, these efforts have also created a new profile of the typical woman in less-developed countries most likely to use infant formula—a woman imagined as poor, urban, poorly educated, and working outside the home.[12]

Yet, in my view, the ways in which infant formula use can contribute to infant death and disease in the global south primarily hinge on infrastructure and economic problems. Without access to clean water or the means to boil water, infant formula made with contaminated water poses a threat to infants. According to UNICEF estimates, children living in places with poor sanitation and no access to safe water are six to twenty-five times more likely to die from diarrheal disease (2007). Without access to adequate wages, mothers dilute formula to stretch it until they can afford to buy more or use complementary but nutritionally inadequate foods, such as rice gruel, to supplement the child's diet.[13] These practices can lead to malnutrition, which in turn renders infants more susceptible to disease and death. In Europe and North America, the use of infant formula does not routinely lead to infant death and disease because most mothers have access to clean water and adequate amounts of formula.[14] While many would consider the use of infant formula less than ideal under any circumstances, we know that it can be and has been a safe means of nourishing infants.[15]

Despite awareness that structural problems contribute to higher rates of infant mortality and disease, interventions undertaken to reduce them continue to target individual mothers and generally neglect the larger structural forces that make infant formula use so risky and breastfeeding unmanageable. The long-standing public-health-oriented strategy to protect infant health thus continues to focus on mothers to increase rates of exclusive breastfeeding. If women followed WHO recommendations to breastfeed exclusively, with no supplements of food or formula for six months, breastfeeding might be, as the epigraph at the beginning of this section states, an inexpensive lifesaver.[16] This logic frames breastfeeding as an exclusively biological rather than social form of reproductive behavior. If we incorporate the social aspects of reproduction into the equation of how best to feed infants, the potential costs to mothers appear. How might exclusive breastfeeding for six months, for example, affect a mother's ability to participate in agricultural or wage labor to support her family? What might six months of exclusive breastfeeding mean for the mother's health? How might exclusive breastfeeding influence family and marital relations?

In sum, approaches to decreasing infant mortality around the world rest on inducing mothers to exclusively breastfeed for six months. Such a solution exemplifies the workings of health promotion described in the "Introduction." Children's, and indeed the world's, future potential can best be realized through their mothers' willingness to breastfeed rather than through substantive structural changes that might improve women's access to health care, maternity leave, and fair wages.[17]

Becoming Baby Friendly: Governing Mothers

On a quiet morning in January, Nurse Bai, the professional in charge of breastfeeding education at the Number 35 Hospital, brought out two paperbound books to show me. Their brightly colored green and yellow covers with a line drawing of a mother breastfeeding a contented infant contained the materials for the training course Nurse Bai and Dr. Wang had taken in preparation for transforming the Number 35 to a BFH. Nurse Bai described the training course with enthusiasm.

> The classes were informative. There was a lot to learn in a short time, but many topics in the lectures were also covered in the books so they could be reviewed later. It was very interesting to learn about breastfeeding and the scientific research that has brought new information to us. For example, the research shows that infants who are breastfed are less likely to have colds and ear infections than children who received cow's milk or infant formula. I like learning new things, and there is so much that is changing in medicine. Many of the women who come here have questions about breastfeeding and other things but don't always have time to ask. Now that I offer the [breastfeeding] classes, they have the opportunity to ask questions and get answers that are not based on superstition or traditional ways.

Nurse Bai's keenness for bringing the necessary changes to the Number 35 Hospital continued as we looked at the course books together. The first book, *Establishing a Baby-Friendly Hospital,* was published in Chinese by the Ministry of Health, but the content was provided by UNICEF, WHO, and Wellstart—a US-based consulting firm that promotes breastfeeding and developed the principles and practices that led to the BFHI (Ministry of Health 1992). The eighty-four-page book is organized like a US continuing-medical-education course, with topics, learning objectives, and outlines of key points. After an introduction by the Ministry's Maternal and Child Health Division establishing that the text was provided by UNICEF/WHO, the book's authors exhort personnel involved in maternal and child health to study and learn the steps necessary to create a BFH and promote breastfeeding whenever possible. Nurse Bai recited the ten steps to me as she pointed to a small poster on the wall that also presented these steps to women as they attended breastfeeding education classes.

> There are ten steps that every hospital in the world must accomplish to become certified as a Baby-Friendly Hospital. First, the hospital must have a written breastfeeding policy that is communicated to all hospital staff. Second, the hospital must train all personnel to implement the policy. Third, all women who receive prenatal care must receive information on the benefits and management of breastfeeding. Fourth, all mothers must be assisted in initiating breastfeeding in the first half hour after childbirth. Fifth, the hospital must educate mothers about how to breastfeed and how to manage the process when away from their infants. Sixth, newborns must not receive any drinks except breast milk unless medically indicated. Seventh, all infants must stay in the room with their mothers twenty-four hours a day. Eighth, women must be shown how to breastfeed on demand. Ninth, there must be no use of artificial nipples or pacifiers for infants. Tenth, the establishment of breastfeeding support groups must be encouraged and mothers referred to them when they are discharged from the hospital. These steps are required by the Ministry of Health, UNICEF, and the WHO [if a hospital is] to receive certification as a Baby-Friendly Hospital.

Much as the placard at the front door of the Number 35 Hospital announced its baby-friendly status, the posting of the ten steps on the wall of the breastfeeding classroom and Nurse Bai's recitation of the steps and her training at a UNICEF/WHO-sponsored course on implementing the BFHI indicate how national and international interests in breastfeeding have come to be incorporated into the spaces and practices of the obstetrics clinic. At the same time, these rather mundane markers of the program's presence in the Number 35 also help to situate the hospital in a larger web of institutions that seek to govern the conduct of new mothers.

Nurse Bai's enthusiasm for the course and the process of becoming a BFH outweighed, in her mind, the problems associated with ensuring that the program requirements were met. When asked whether there were difficulties in establishing and maintaining the ten steps, she replied:

> Some of the difficulties our hospital faced were that we had to reorganize some staff responsibilities. Since we would no longer keep infants in a nursery, those nurses had to be reassigned to take care of women on the obstetrics ward or they had the option of working in the pediatrics ward. These nurses were not happy about these changes. Other nursing staff were concerned that having infants with their mothers on the wards would mean more work for them since they would not have scheduled times to help the mothers when the infants were delivered to them every two to three hours for feeding as in the past. Instead they worried that other work would be constantly interrupted by mothers asking for help with their infants. One nurse said that she might be distracted from other patient care tasks if mothers had their infants with them all the time. It is true that the wards are noisy now that the babies are staying with their mothers—there is little privacy, and if one infant cries, everyone must listen to it. . . . Another problem is that it is difficult to oversee the advice and practices that older female relatives give the new mothers. Sometimes they will bring in bottles and formulas or sugar water if they think the infant needs it. It can be difficult to monitor these things when you are busy, but most of the time, after you explain why it is

> not good for the baby to have a bottle, they listen. But I am an older woman myself, and people tend to listen to me. Some of the younger nurses have a hard time convincing older people to take their advice.

Nurse Bai looked up at the list of the ten steps and commented, "We don't really have any breastfeeding support groups, but all women are visited at home at least once after their discharge. That is the best we can do right now." Nurse Bai's description of her experiences with establishing a BFH show that she was aware of, and in further conversation, excited about, participating in a multilateral program. She noted, "We are part of an international program, and China is taking this very seriously; this will help raise the quality of China's population and its development and strength." In one of the training manuals, a section is devoted to teaching health professionals the history of breastfeeding promotion at the WHO. Nurse Bai, who was unaware of this history prior to her training, suggested that China had been concerned with supporting breastfeeding long before the BFHI.

> China, as a poor country, supported breastfeeding by giving women breaks during the workday to breastfeed and providing paid maternity leaves. This was a government policy for a long time, but things have changed now. There were few good substitutes for breast milk, and it was more practical for families and the government to encourage breastfeeding. It was not easy in those days [when she was herself] a breastfeeding and working mother]. Now, however, a lot of work units do not want to hire married women who have not yet had children as they are considered less efficient and more trouble. Everything is about making money, and giving women breaks to breastfeed during the day means the company loses her labor for that time. . . . Other companies and work units try to get women to take a long maternity leave and pay them only half their salaries because they can hire someone without children who will work for less money and fewer benefits. So, although I think the Baby-Friendly Hospital is a good idea, there are pressures on women in the workplace that the hospital cannot really change. Other policies and changes must be made by the government to actually increase breastfeeding in China.

Nurse Bai echoes the issue raised in the pamphlet discussed earlier in the Introduction about the difficulties women face as they balance work and infant feeding. She is aware that the BFHI cannot change the pressures that women experience if they try to work full time and breastfeed. Additionally, as she describes the problems and concerns encountered during the process of becoming a BFH, it becomes clear that while professional expertise is essential to the program it may also be undermined when infants, no longer kept in a separate nursery, require nurses to negotiate new terrain in the obstetrics ward. Nurse Bai also notes that China had made serious attempts in the past to support breastfeeding for working women so that in her eyes the BFHI is part of a long historical effort on the state's part to ensure the well-being of its future generations. In all, her reactions provide a glimpse of some of the assumptions built into the practical aspects of program implementation.

Nurse Bai's recounting of the course on the BFHI, the steps taken at the Number 35 Hospital to become baby friendly, and China's previous policies to promote breastfeeding outline the contours of a new form of maternal governance. Much as the state opened its doors to foreign investment and consumer goods, the implementation of the BFHI opened the door to embracing global standards and strategies to increase breastfeeding among its citizen-mothers. Reactions to these assumptions and the program are taken up in later chapters in more detail. For now exploration of how the BFHI fits into China's political and social agendas can help set part of the stage for understanding the constraints and opportunities the thirty women in this study faced, as well as the ways in which the program relied on biological reasoning within the confines of a BFH in Beijing.

The National Mother and Citizen-Child

As Nurse Bai suggested, China's commitment to breastfeeding has been remarkable. Its number-one ranking in the world for creating BFHs marks a continuation of widespread and long-standing efforts to promote breastfeeding (Xinhua News Agency 1996b). In the 1970s it was one of the few countries to adhere to the guidelines of the

International Labor Organization (ILO) in support of breastfeeding among working women by providing two nursing breaks during the workday along with extended maternity leave (Pasternak and Wang 1985). Importantly, the ILO policies were implemented prior to the economic reforms initiated in 1978 and the importation of western brands of breast milk substitutes beginning in 1985. Despite these efforts, the number of urban mothers who breastfed for six months declined from 81 percent in 1950 to less than 11 percent in 1992 (*China Daily*, August 8, 92). To address this dramatic decline, the Chinese government worked with WHO/UNICEF and designed policies and laws to promote breastfeeding as part of a more comprehensive program to improve child health by the year 2000 (Xinhua News Agency 1996b). As spaces and routines in maternity wards and clinics were reorganized, obstetrics personnel attended workshops and classes that taught practical techniques for working with new mothers and infants. For example, Nurse Bai, the breastfeeding educator, and Dr. Wang, a pediatrician at the Number 35, were among more than eight hundred thousand physicians, nurses, and other health workers in China who were trained to convince new mothers that breastfeeding was a better choice than infant formula and to help them learn how to breastfeed (Yuan 1997).[18] At one level, the spatial reorganization of the Number 35 Hospital represented the results of interplay between international and national policy agendas that seek to attain the stated goal of reversing breastfeeding declines. On another level, it offered Chinese medical workers an opportunity to reexamine hospital organization and concrete health care practices in light of national and international standards. Further, the process represents an example of how the new public health described earlier works. But most important, at the heart of these reforms stand the mother and her infant. The Chinese state's renewed focus on maternal and child health—bolstered by the BFHI—at once reinforced state interest in women's reproductive lives and created possibilities for women as citizen-mothers to make decisions about how best to rear their single child in a rapidly changing China.

The flurry of attention to maternal and child health in the early 1990s is evident in the number of United Nations programs, laws, and policies adopted by China's leaders. For example, Premier Li Peng signed the World Declaration on the Survival, Protection, and Development of Children, as well as the Plan of Action for Implementing the World Declaration on the Survival, Protection, and Development of Children, after China participated in the United Nations World Summit for Children in 1990. In addition, China cosponsored the draft resolution for the United Nations Convention on the Rights of Children, which was formally approved in 1991 and adopted by the Chinese government in 1992 (Xinhua News Agency 1996b). This was preceded by the ratification in 1980 of the United Nations Convention on the Elimination of All Forms of Discrimination against Women (CEDAW).[19] Such state-sponsored actions mark important instances in which the Chinese government accepted international standards and goals regarding maternal and child health and signaled its willingness to conform to international law in certain realms.[20] This participation partly stemmed from Chinese leaders' understanding that to be considered on a par and to compete with other developed countries the nation must raise its living standards and improve the health and well-being of its citizens. Healthy infants become sturdy citizens of a strong state.

China's engagement with these multilateral initiatives reinforced the legitimacy and urgency in official discourse in the early to mid-1990s where clear links were made between the importance of children in the state's plans to improve the overall population and the ultimate well-being of the nation. For example, a white paper issued by China's State Council states, "Children's survival, protection, and development, which are the basis for improving the quality of the population and the prerequisite conditions for the advance of mankind, directly concern a country and a nation's future and destiny" (Xinhua News Agency 1996b). Most relevant to this study is how the state planned to achieve these goals. Later in the report, improving child nutrition through breastfeeding stands alongside such factors as improving access to education and medical care and protecting disabled and orphaned children. The presence of breastfeeding in the report reinforces China's embrace of the BFHI but also brings into focus a specific maternal behavior as a target for oversight and change. Education and medical care, by contrast, require the efforts of multiple stakeholders—from parents to educators to physicians.

The document also reminds readers of the state's power to improve the quality of births by legal means. Referring to a 1994–95 law protecting maternal and child health, the report notes, "This law is formulated according to the Constitution to guarantee the health of mothers and infants by improving the quality of births" (Xinhua News Agency 1996b). The rhetorical importance of the mother is signified only as the means of producing an infant. The subsequent quality of potential children is emphasized most clearly in the extensive sections of the law addressing health care during pregnancy and childbirth. Essentially, the law requires the supervision of conception, pregnancy, and the postpartum period by medical personnel in the interest of producing healthy, physically normal infants. The law specifies that in any situation in which the potential for abnormality of the fetus exists as the result of hereditary conditions, lifestyle, or other disease, health care providers may intervene and determine the necessity of terminating the pregnancy.[21] Mothers are invisible as agents in these state-produced documents and at least at this level of discourse are relegated to the status of vessels through which the nation can reproduce and develop. The tenor of these Chinese policies is not unique. Allison Jagger, in her study of reproduction and the body, observes that in most cultures pregnant women "are viewed less as individuals than as the 'raw material' from which the 'product' is extracted. In modern [western] circumstances it is possible to understand how the physician rather than the mother comes to be seen as having produced the baby" (1983, 311).[22]

The interests of the Chinese state in this instance mesh with the logic and assumptions underlying health promotion or the new public health, as discussed earlier, with regard to the WHO and UNICEF. Underlying these multilateral programs, national laws, and policies is a biological notion of citizenship.[23] From the one-child policy to the BFHI, reproduction was considered the biological foundation of China's future in the 1990s. Susan Greenhalgh (2008), drawing on Foucault's concept of biopolitics, shows how reproduction is subject to state-organized scrutiny and regulation, which are carried out for a variety of strategic purposes essential to governance.[24] The state, then, in the collective interests of the nation, can legitimately regulate and control reproduction. In this case, deputizing medical professionals and organizations like BFHs serves to minimize risks to society and individuals in the interest of producing a healthy populace.[25] The state achieves this goal in the case of infant feeding by singling out the individual mother and focusing on policies and practices that aim to shape her behavior. Mothers in Chinese law and policy continue to operate as vehicles for reproduction, and consequently the state's authority subsumes their autonomy and interests (Greenhalgh and Winkler 2005). While this conclusion is by no means a new one, these laws protecting children, along with implementation of the BFHI, offer a new mechanism by means of which the state can maintain an interest in reproduction beyond the one-child policy's goal of limiting population growth. The BFHI expands the time frame of government intervention and oversight so that women's postpartum decisions and autonomy also become subject to the state's interest in producing healthy citizens.

However, by the mid-1990s the state's interests began to intersect with those of its citizens. As will become apparent in later chapters, women in my study voiced concerns about the "quality" of their children, not only in relation to national-level goals of improving the nation but also in terms of their desire to participate in a modern lifestyle by limiting family size. It is here that governmentality and a biopolitics of a subtler order come to light. As individuals internalize values about high-quality children, they locate ways to make such values relevant to their own interests. Susan Champagne shows how popular books on child rearing in the 1980s and 1990s provided concrete advice on assessing and implementing techniques and technologies to ensure that children would reach their full intellectual potential (1992).

Unlike the still strict one-child policy in the mid-1990s, the tactic used by the BFHI sought to reinforce or reshape individual women's aspirations and desires, as well as playing on their anxiety for their children's future at a time of rapid social and economic change.[26] And among a number of women their interests and that of the BFHI did coincide. Women like Sun Li, a twenty-eight-year-old factory worker, made comments, including this one, on a few occasions in our first meetings.

> I want to be sure that my infant is as healthy, strong, and intelligent as possible, and I have learned that breastfeeding is the best thing I can do for my child. China is changing, and my child will need to be prepared so that he/she can have a good life in the future. It will probably mean some sacrifices; I will probably take a longer maternity leave than I would like. [She then laughed and said] We will try not to, but we will probably rely on her/him to help us!

Much as Sun Li believed the best thing she could do would be to take a longer leave from work in order to breastfeed her newborn, other women, as we will see in the next chapter, were not so certain that breastfeeding was the best way to ensure a healthy, intelligent child. Thus, despite intersecting interests, such protectionist policies created new dilemmas for Chinese women.[27] Indirect forms of governmentality, like that of the BFHI, may work as they are intended, but there are always unintended outcomes and other possible responses to these efforts.

Black Cat, White Cat: The Practical Mother

Chinese leader Deng Xiaoping famously stated, "It does not matter whether it is a black cat or a white cat. If it catches mice, it is a good cat."[28] His remark signified the importance of adopting a pragmatic rather than political approach to China's economic and social development. Much as Deng advocated practical approaches to change, China's rapid economic growth brought about three linked transformations for women in the 1990s that shaped their experiences in the BFH. The state relaxed a number of economic policies, including its hold on state-owned enterprises. It allowed the development of private companies, small businesses, and foreign-Chinese joint ventures;

opened the country to more imported goods; and enacted new laws and policies protecting women's employment. These changes helped bring about the unprecedented availability of consumer goods, from clothing, food products, televisions, and washing machines to everything in between, and ushered in a new consumer-oriented culture. Shopping at newly renovated department stores and bookstores, drinking in teahouses, and eating in restaurants became new leisure activities. However, these changes also brought increasing uncertainty in women's employment. State enterprises, for example, no longer subsidized by government funding, had to make a profit to become self-sustaining. One key way to cut costs and increase efficiency was to eliminate jobs, and as a result the women in this study were concerned about keeping their jobs after the birth of their children. We will see that women navigated between the demands of motherhood and their employment situations beginning in pregnancy to ensure some measure of security.

The issue of women's public contributions has been a key one for the Chinese state, even when national employment problems and economic policies took precedence over the goal of giving women access to full employment opportunities (Andors 1983). Thus, the state's messages about women inevitably contain dual images of their proper role as worker and mother at any given moment, and the 1990s were no different. The 1992 Rights and Protection of Women Law, for example, aims to protect women workers during their reproductive years. Specifically, Articles 26 and 27 sustain the dual roles of women.

> Article 26. All units shall, in line with women's characteristics and according to law, protect women's safety and health during their work or physical labour, and shall not assign them any work or physical labour not suitable to women. Women shall be under special protection during [their] menstrual period, pregnancy, obstetrical period and nursing period.
>
> Article 27. No unit shall reduce the salaries or wages of female workers and staff members, or dismiss them, or unilaterally cancel the labour (or employment) contracts or service agreements with

> them because they are married, pregnant, on maternity leave or breast-feeding, except where female workers and staff members request termination of the labour (or employment) contracts or service agreements themselves.[29]

Despite the law's intentions, its representation of women as mothers or potential mothers first and workers second provided reinforcement for employers and enterprises wishing to avoid hiring fertile women in the first place.[30]

Official concerns regarding the effect of the economic reforms on family life also reinforce contradictory messages about women in Chinese society. For example, a 1980s official campaign urging women to act as "virtuous wives and good mothers" highlights a thread of rhetoric that continued in the 1990s (and into the twenty-first century), suggesting that women should be relegated to special roles in the work force based on their physiological differences or should consider becoming housewives (Feng Bian 1984 quoted in Honig and Hershatter 1988).[31] In spite of its increasingly capitalist orientation, the Chinese government continues to view itself as morally bound to reinforce and promote values it considers paramount for the country's social and national welfare.

While many women in this study sought to balance their work and family lives, they were also participating in the expanding consumer culture in Beijing. Two aspects of this culture were particularly evident in the 1990s and are especially relevant because they contradicted the state's emphasis on women as conforming to an ideal of mothers who breastfed their children. First, women were making infant feeding decisions at a moment of dramatic growth in the production, marketing, and sales of baby foods, an industry that rapidly expanded beginning in the mid-1980s. Second, new products designed to enhance female beauty and the sexualized portrayal of women's bodies in media productions created another level of anxiety and desire for new mothers at a particularly vulnerable time in their lives.

Sales of baby foods in China reached US$37.1 million in 1995 and $12 billion in 2008 (Harney 2013). Foreign companies, such as Nestle and Borden, led the market in this industry in China (Eurofood 1996, 3). The availability of commercial, foreign infant formula represented China's success in its economic reforms and opening to international trade. Yet the sale of infant formula runs counter to the BFHI's goal of increasing breastfeeding rates. These competing forces, the pressure to breastfeed and pressure to use formula, met head on in the Number 35 Hospital and affected women's infant feeding choices. As will become apparent in later chapters, among the women who chose to use infant formula, the majority justified their decisions using the same images and constructs of science and modernity as those promoted in the BFHI.

The extent of China's official commitment to promoting breastfeeding is evident in its passage of the 1995 National Provisions on Marketing of Breast Milk Substitutes Law. It regulates the marketing and selling of infant formula to women in hospitals. China joined more than 118 countries that have adopted the principles of the 1981 international WHO Code to stop the deceptive marketing practices of infant formula companies in developing countries (Maher 1992). This Code's ten provisions limit the marketing of breast milk substitutes, cereals, teas, and bottles and includes the following restrictions: no advertising of any products to the public; no free samples given to mothers; no promotion of products in health care facilities, including the distribution of free or low-cost supplies; no company sales representatives to advise mothers; no gifts or personal samples given to health workers; and no words or pictures idealizing artificial feeding or pictures of infants on labels of infant milk containers. The code warns that information given to health workers must be scientific and factual, all information on artificial infant feeding must explain the benefits of breastfeeding and the costs and hazards associated with infant formula, and nutritionally unsuitable products such as sweetened condensed milk must not be promoted for babies.[32]

At the same time that this law was adopted in China, the attractions of foreign investment and profit seeking overcame the state's reluctance to allow the production and promotion of infant formula. Profits available to firms making breast milk substitutes are high; Mead Johnson's 1996 annual report indicated that Enfamil (a breast milk substitute) was listed as one of its "high growth products," having experienced a 24 percent increase in sales worldwide, and was considered the company's third-best-selling product (*Mead Johnson Annual Report,* 1996). China, with its vast population and nearly 20 million births every year (China Statistical Bureau 1994), represented and continues to represent a huge potential market for infant formula. In 1994–96, three foreign companies and a myriad of Chinese firms dominated the formula industry in China.[33] In fact, one report notes that Mead Johnson formed the Mead Johnson (Guangzhou) Co. Ltd. joint venture to produce and package infant milk products with a total investment of US$30 million, 85 percent of which was financed by the US company (Stevenson-Yang 1996). This market, despite a number of instances of widespread tainted infant formula in China, continues to expand. By 2012 infant formula accounted for more than US$13.3 billion in sales to Chinese consumers (Harney 2013).

Furthermore, during my fieldwork I witnessed the promotion of nutritional drink products to mothers during and after pregnancy by foreign formula companies, presumably to establish brand loyalty if the mother decided to use infant formula. Mead Johnson marketed a product called MaMa Sustagen for pregnant and nursing women in Beijing. Since the product is not technically an infant formula, the company was and continues to be allowed to market it in hospitals and through representatives. By 2014 most infant formula companies had developed a maternal nutritional drink powder and were also manufacturing prenatal vitamins.

The contradiction between the state's adoption of the international code to limit the sale and marketing of breast milk substitutes as a means of promoting breastfeeding on the one hand and the development of joint ventures to produce infant formula on the other, speaks to the conflicting realities women face when they choose their infant feeding method. While the state promotes the idea that breastfeeding is the best way to feed an infant, it also has an interest in providing high-quality alternatives that bring profit and investment to China. This tension between the promotion of child health by increasing breastfeeding and the pressures of economic development that faced China in the 1990s reflected, at a macrolevel, the contradictions inherent in conceptions of Chinese women's lives. In addition, the promotion of nutritional drinks for pregnant and nursing women created an additional structure of authority for defining ideals of motherhood and mothering. Using the rhetoric and concerns articulated by state policies and authorities, these types of products represented maternal nutrition as a condition that at once required intervention and women's compliant behavior. As we will see in chapter 2, these contradictory approaches were played out in the hospital setting, where mothers were taught how to feed their infants. In the meantime, this brief sketch serves as a reminder that the forms of biogovernance by the Chinese state at times compete with or contradict other national agendas.

The Feminine Mother

As urban Chinese men and women became consumers and producers in the global market, the social, symbolic, and experiential aspects of gender identity were, and would continue in the twenty-first century, to change. In the 1980s, public and private discourse centered on issues such as relationships, beauty, women's work, sexuality, and divorce. These discussions represented a rejection of the uniformity of experience and material life imposed during the Cultural Revolution (Honig and Hershatter 1988; Robinson 1985). The mid-1990s were characterized by a deepening engagement with global economic and cultural forces that reinforced these concerns. Later in the book, I link the ways the explosion in the marketing and consumption of beauty and fashion products in urban China in the 1990s precipitated a new conception of the ideal feminine body and how new mothers negotiated and created a sense of self in this context. For now, however, I want to highlight the larger-scale dynamics of consumerism and the feminine body. Susan Bordo's (1993) reflection on the body seems apt for beginning a discussion on the relations between these two phenomena. Bordo expands on Mary Douglas's observation that rigid bodily boundaries maintained by rules and rituals are most often found in societies whose external boundaries are weak or under attack (Douglas 1986, 114–28). Bordo suggests, "Let me hypothesize, similarly, that preoccupation with the 'internal' management of the body (that is management of its desires) is produced by instabilities in what could be called the macro-regulation of desire within the system of the social body" (1993, 199). With its economic and social boundaries in a great deal of flux in the early to mid-1990s, desires at the macro- and individual levels were manifested in ideas about how to best manage the female body (Rofel 2007).

Indeed, a new preoccupation with sexuality as a form of consumer desire in this milieu gave rise to emphases on the feminine body as both a marker of modernity and a site of self-management. It was difficult to ignore the plethora of beauty magazines sold on street corners or the myriad counters of cosmetic products in department stores throughout Beijing. Chinese women, in their roles as wives and mothers, encountered ways of being requiring attention to their sexuality and attractiveness as a part of their identity formation. While in many ways these changes contrast with earlier socialist ideals that emphasized women's contribution to the socialist collective, these representations maintain a convergence and similarity that presupposes women are the essential caretakers of the domestic sphere (Evans 1997, 142).[34] These dynamics have continued in the twenty-first century as women are still portrayed, in popular cultural representations found in magazines, television advertisements, and most recently Internet sites, as the primary actors in maintaining a felicitous and well-managed family life.

Systematic studies of representations of women in Chinese media in the 1990s reinforced my impressions and observations of this phenomenon. In a survey that examined 1,197 television commercials broadcast over a five-month period, researchers found that women were portrayed as housewives (51.5 percent of the time) and when female characters were depicted in the workplace their concerns centered on "their withering hair, or feeling uneasy about their menstrual period. Otherwise they are shown to be thinking of an upcoming date" (Lei 1997, 2).[35] That women were represented in the housewife role when in China more than 70 percent of women over the age of fifteen work outside the home represents an important disconnection between the ideals and reality of gender roles. The message conveyed by such advertising is that the home and family life are the purview of modern women. Furthermore, young, attractive women played 87 percent of the female roles in these commercials, which presupposed that beauty and femininity sell products (2). These findings may not seem surprising to western readers, but they reflected an increasingly consumer-oriented culture in which advertisers sought to attract customers using gender stereotypes and roles and promoting the notion that modernity, success, and happiness can be achieved through consumption.

These representations only begin to illuminate the intersection of consumerism and female identity. A study based on twelve thousand households in Heilongjiang Province found that individuals were spending increasing amounts of money on clothing and makeup. In 1991 per capita expenditures on clothing reached US$44 (231.45 Yuan), an increase of 60.3 percent since 1987, and expenditures on cosmetics were 1.2 times higher than in 1987 (Zheng 1992). The increases in consumer spending on these types of products demonstrated that people were paying more attention to their personal appearance. While the statistics do not break down spending by gender, sales of cosmetics and other product targeted at female consumers continued to grow. Color cosmetics, which include facial and nail products, accounted for 6 percent of the personal care product expenditures made by Chinese consumers in 1993 and was considered to be the fastest-growing sector of this market niche (Swanson 1995, 34). Availability of these items simply exploded in the mid-1990s. For example, with more than seven hundred cosmetics on sale at a department store in Harbin, Chinese women could find and purchase any number of beauty products (37). These trends have continued. By 2012 foreign cosmetics companies, from Avon and Mary Kay to Estee Lauder and Shiseido, accounted for 80 percent of the market. These top international brands posted US$17.3 billion (107.7 billion yuan) in sales to Chinese consumers in 2012 (State of Israel Ministry of Trade 2012). Advertising, consumption, and production patterns of beauty products illustrate the increasing importance of personal appearance to young Chinese women and marked a change from the 1970s. But, as we will learn from the women in this study, they also played into more complex dynamics about the conflation of sex appeal and marital sexual relations, on the one hand, and the happy homemaker and mother on the other. Ultimately these new possibilities for consumption and shaping women's identities represent another facet of potentiality and a new form of governance. Women's decisions about whether and how to adopt or adapt to these new demands would have far-reaching consequences for the stability of their marriages and families.

Conclusion

In the mid-1990s, the hospital operated as one location where women from pregnancy through the postpartum period came into contact with the ideals of femininity and body image that formed a part of consumer desires in post-reform China. Paradoxically, it was there, in the very spaces that persuade women to breastfeed, that these messages about beauty predominated. However, it was not only international firms that advertised their products; local companies also played to the idealized fit and trim body that urban Chinese popular culture promoted in the 1990s. The sexually attractive breastfeeding mother found on posters, book covers, and advertisements reveals the contradictory discursive and experiential contexts that women confronted as they assimilated the role of motherhood into their identities and made infant feeding decisions. This unique moment deserves attention, for it was a time when women underwent bodily changes beyond their immediate control in a cultural and social milieu that encouraged self-control and regulation as a means of achieving the ideal, feminine body. The arrival of new forms of maternal governance through consumer culture and laws and policies like the BFH provided a site where it is possible to see these processes at work.

Beyond these institutional forces, individual women, as they embarked on the road to becoming a mother to a single child, confronted the ideals, traditions, and practices of a society that emphasized the importance of children in terms of the family and its future. The result of these multiple messages was often contradictory or at times represented an unattainable ideal—the sexually attractive and available breastfeeding mother of an only child. In the chapters that follow, we will see how the intersection of governmental and cultural influences on gender formation influenced women as they became mothers and made decisions about how best to nourish their children.

CHAPTER TWO

Nature and Science

Making Modern Mothers in the Baby Friendly Hospital

Introduction

The choice of a hospital as a site for educating women about infant feeding has a checkered history. Since the 1950s, urban hospitals in many parts of the world have discouraged breastfeeding because the established routines and practices of maternity wards separate mothers and infants except during scheduled feeding times.[1] With increasing worldwide interest in promoting breastfeeding in the late 1970s to reduce infant disease and mortality in the global south, researchers discovered that more than routine separation of mothers and babies in hospitals influenced infant feeding practices. Hospitals allowing distribution of free infant formula samples resulted in new mothers associating the formula with medicine and thus a "modern" and "scientific" product (Jelliffe and Jelliffe 1978). Other findings have shown that hospital professionals often have little knowledge of or training in breastfeeding. As a result, they can convey negative attitudes supported by their medical authority.[2] This research reflects broader developments in health promotion that sought to account for the role of external factors in shaping individual health behavior. By the early 1990s, hospitals came to be viewed by public health policy makers as key locations where a variety of messages, practices, and role models were likely influencing women's infant feeding practices.

The women in this study arrived at the Number 35 Hospital for the breastfeeding classes from worlds where they were pregnant with their only child in accordance with state policy; where they faced the expectation of family members that they would produce a healthy, intelligent grandchild; and where they faced growing uncertainty about their future employment. These women also navigated an increasingly capitalist and consumer-oriented society where value was placed on individuality and choice. They also found themselves encountering new expectations of femininity and sexuality. Evans observed in the 1990s, "Practices of body management, long and obsessively publicized in Western societies, are now prominent in the Chinese media. How to cultivate beautiful pale skin, exercise to keep the body slim and supple and massage to keep breasts in shape are all familiar topics in women's magazines" (1997, 140). However, the bodily imperatives found in popular media did not reflect the physical experiences of women during and after pregnancy.

Paradoxically, in the BFH the flawless, sexualized female body appeared in both state-produced images and messages that endorsed breastfeeding and in international infant formula manufacturers' promotional literature. As noted in the "Introduction," both entities played on women's concerns with bodily management in the discourse used to ally their products (infant formula) or practices (breastfeeding) with the cachet of modernity and cosmopolitanism (See figs. 1 and 2). Further, infant formula companies drew on the state's rhetoric and ideals about producing a healthy future generation. Women were encouraged to sustain bodies capable of breastfeeding their infants as part of their duty to adhere to larger state policies and produce a healthy population. Yet they also encountered sexualized ideals of a slim body in the hospital's promotion of breastfeeding. The discourse of the BFHI and infant formula companies thus drew on collective concerns with the health and future

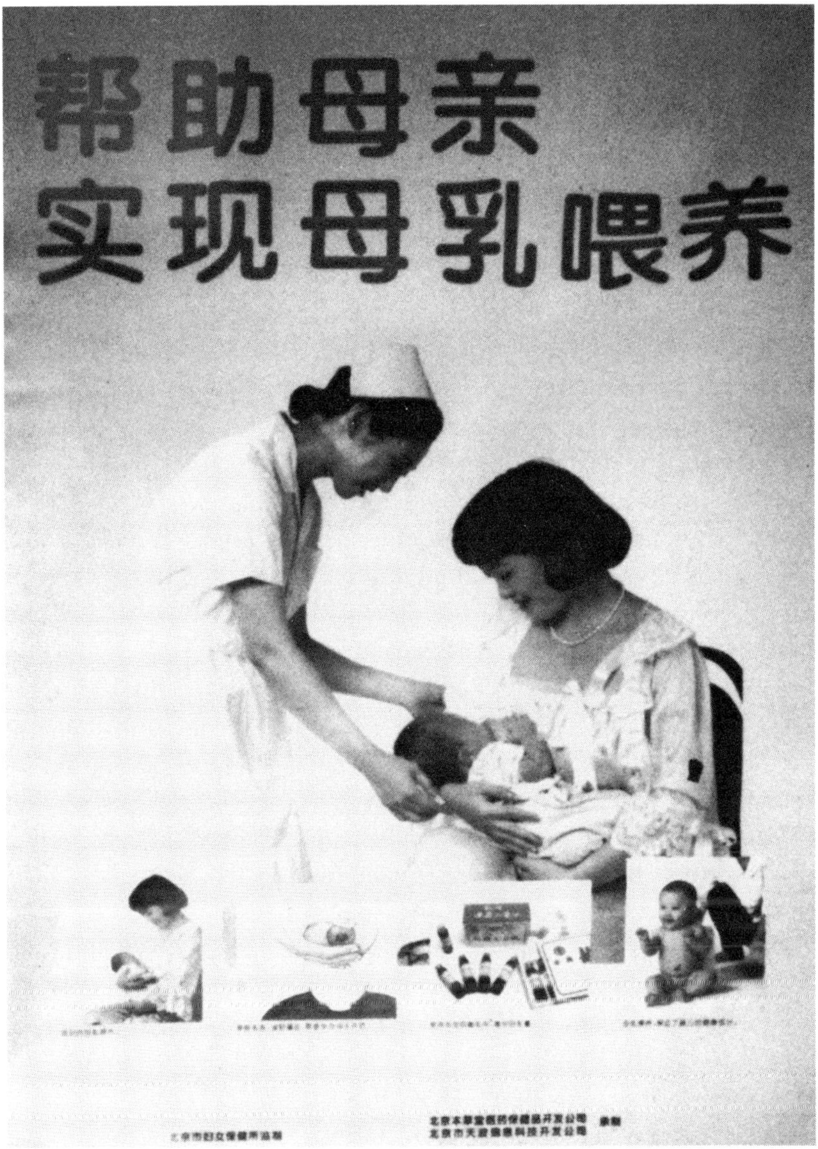

Figure 2. Poster in the hallway of the obstetrics clinic

of the nation and on women's individual interests in nourishing their infants and managing their bodies. These tensions reflected what was happening outside the walls of the Number 35 Hospital in the mid-1990s.

The Number 35 Hospital grounded the manifestations of these complex and often contradictory changes in its spaces—the hallways, clinics, and waiting areas—as well as among the people who worked in and visited the obstetrics clinic. The hospital might be usefully understood as a locale made up of a constellation of relations that brought the social and cultural dynamics particular to the Number 35 into contact with large-scale social relations, processes, and understandings. These constellations thus also embodied the potentiality of reproduction and the potentiality of consumer culture within and outside the hospital walls. As a result these spaces were also likely to be locations of internal differences and conflicts (Massey 1993, 66). This chapter offers an ethnographic perspective on the ways, in a Chinese hospital, meanings of modernity and science blurred the lines between state imperatives to produce national subjects and citizens and the flexibility accorded to individual women through their participation in more transnational economies of capitalism. We also see how the intersection of local, national, and transnational representations that result from these constellations of relations worked to shape women's experiences in contradictory ways as they participated in their prenatal health care and anticipated how to best feed their infants.[3]

The chapter first follows three women through the mandatory breastfeeding classes where we can see the ways in which the discourse in these sessions drew on medical authority and expert knowledge, modernity and science, femininity, and citizenship to persuade women that "breast is best." From these sessions, we look in more depth at how the dialectic of nature and science in promoting breastfeeding became complicated when Nurse Bai made a pragmatic decision to distribute advertising pamphlets for prenatal nutritional drinks that also promoted the product lines of infant formula companies. The chapter then turns to focus on how women responded to the often conflicting messages about women's bodies and infant feeding that appeared in the class materials sanctioned by the BFHI, the infant formula company pamphlets, and the posters dotting the hallway of the obstetrics clinic. In discussions about weight gain and loss, exercise, beauty, and femininity, we learn how women navigated among the long-standing pressures to produce a healthy infant for family and nation and newer forces that brought ideals of beauty and femininity to bear on the maternal body. It is in these hospital spaces, then, that we see new forms of maternal governance emerging. However, this chapter demonstrates that as much as the policies described in chapter 1 attempted to solve discrete problems for the nation and the international community (through UNICEF and WHO), in practice unanticipated contradictions and convergences complicated the program's potential success in convincing mothers to breastfeed their infants.

Educating Mothers: Breastfeeding Is Best

Images urging women to breastfeed appeared throughout the lobby and first-floor hallways of the Number 35 Hospital, but it was in the Obstetrics and Gynecology Outpatient Clinic that the imprint of the BFHI was most readily apparent. The clinic consisted of a long hallway with rooms off to each side. As they arrived, patients registered at a small desk staffed by a receptionist at one end of the hallway and then waited on wooden folding chairs to be called to one of the two examination rooms. Pregnant women carried their own medical records, which they handed to the receptionist, who charged a small fee for their visit. As these women waited to see the physician, they could not help but notice the numerous images of nursing women and the ubiquitous messages celebrating breastfeeding as the best source of nutrition to produce a mentally and physically healthy child. These posters, however, conveyed more than messages about breastfeeding. Many posters were handmade, consisting of scraps from magazines pasted onto large sheets of construction paper.[4] One poster presented an incongruous message as it featured lobster, corn on the cob, and vegetables as items of a healthy diet—a typical New

England lobster dinner clearly unrelated to the normal diet of anyone in the hospital, including pregnant women.[5] When I asked a clinic nurse what it meant, she explained that the color scheme, bright red, yellow, and green, mattered: "No one thinks they should eat such foods; who has the money? But it has good, strong colors that will help women to notice the message that pregnant women should be aware of their diet. The message is the important aspect." Another large poster announced a breastfeeding hotline for women, and as I wondered how interesting it would be to learn more about the types of issues it handled, Nurse Bai, who was in charge of breastfeeding education, laughed and called it a "cold line" (*liang xian*) with a telephone number that had been transferred out of her unit to another part of the hospital. No one had bothered to take down the sign. At the end of the hallway, the room used for prenatal breastfeeding education was furnished with a small desk, a cabinet, benches, a television, and a videocassette recorder (VCR). Posters and a framed set of texts outlining the rules and regulations of the BFHI lined the walls of the room. This classroom, the hallway, and the examination rooms formed the spatial context in which all pregnant women planning to deliver their babies at the hospital confronted and navigated the multiple and intertwined messages and practices associated with the BFHI.

As a part of the BFHI, women were required to attend three breastfeeding classes during pregnancy, beginning with their third- or fourth-month checkup and again at seven and nine months. I use the term *breastfeeding class,* but the Number 35 Hospital did not in fact schedule meetings; Nurse Bai conducted ad hoc sessions as women arrived in the room. Women attended prenatal checkups in the obstetrics clinic on a first-come, first-served basis—there were no appointments or schedules. Without any way to anticipate when a group of women might have been available to form a class, a constant flow of women in and out of the room during morning clinic hours often resulted in a variety of activities simultaneously occurring as part of the breastfeeding education program. Before we look at the sessions more closely, I offer a detailed description of the information presented to women and the ways in which Nurse Bai approached them in this environment. The following cases are representative of sessions I observed over the course of twelve months.

Session One: Introducing Breastfeeding

Nurse Bai greets Li Yurong, a twenty-four-year-old office worker, and asks her to sit on the bench and submit her receipt for payment for the class (three Yuan or about forty cents). She records her name, age, and anticipated date of delivery, along with the date and time of the first class, in a lined notebook. Once the record-keeping details are completed, Nurse Bai tells Li Yurong that as part of her prenatal care she will be attending three sessions where they will discuss the importance of breastfeeding, practice breastfeeding and other infant care techniques (with a doll), and address any of Li's own concerns.

In a conversational tone, Nurse Bai begins with a brief summary of the benefits of breastfeeding.

> Breastfeeding is the best nutrition for your precious one (*baobao*); it has special qualities that cannot be found in infant formula or milk powder. There is scientific evidence showing that breast milk contains things that improve a baby's immune system and brain development. So you can protect your infant from getting sick—especially things like ear infections and colds. It also saves time washing bottles and money; infant formula can be expensive, especially the foreign brands. These days everything is getting more expensive, but you can provide the best for your infant without spending money on infant formula. It saves time, especially at night! You won't have to get out of bed and prepare a bottle for your baby. Breastfeeding creates a bond between mother and infant. This bond is important for the baby's psychological development and physical development, too. Some women worry that they might not have enough milk, but all women, except those that have unique issues, can provide enough breast milk for their infants. You should give your infant only breast milk until it is four months old; then you may start to slowly add other foods. Breast

milk is also natural! It is the best way to feed your baby so it will grow into an intelligent child.

Nurse Bai then turns her attention to Li Yurong's body, asking her to lift her shirt. She then examines Li's breasts while demonstrating how to massage and wash them to prepare for the act of nursing. After practicing with Nurse Bai, Li Yurong is told to massage her breasts and nipples two times a day throughout the pregnancy. This portion of the session takes about ten minutes.

After Nurse Bai completes the massage lesson, she asks Li Yurong if she has any questions, to which Li Yurong replies that she understands everything. Finally, Nurse Bai tells Li Yurong about the importance of good nutrition during her pregnancy and hands her a glossy, full-color pamphlet outlining pregnant women's nutritional needs published by a western formula company that advertises a nutritional supplement for pregnant women.[6] Nurse Bai explains that the pamphlet contains important information but Li Yurong does not need to buy the supplement; she should simply eat a balanced diet to satisfy her nutritional needs.[7] During this session, Li Yurong is not talkative, and Nurse Bai doesn't attempt to engage in conversation beyond her instructional obligations. I found that, while the content of the instruction varied little between encounters, the interpersonal dynamic between Nurse Bai and the pregnant women did: some women initiated conversation while others were silent, responding only to direct questions. In situations where women did not engage, Nurse Bai dominated and used more didactic teaching methods. The first session contained little practical information about breastfeeding and, as Nurse Bai pointed out to me, aimed to introduce women to the idea and benefits of breastfeeding. She felt it was important to first explain the significance of breastfeeding and wait until women are farther along in their pregnancies to discuss more practical elements, such as proper positioning techniques, management of milk production, and especially engorgement. When asked why she handed out informational pamphlets produced by foreign formula companies—a seeming contradiction to her messages about breastfeeding—she noted her concern: "Young women today may not realize the importance of good nutrition during pregnancy.[8] Everyone is busy, and especially early in pregnancy, many women experience upset stomachs and vomiting, so they avoid eating properly." She said that the hospital did not have pamphlets of its own and the formula companies representatives gave them to her free of charge. She acknowledged that these companies "advertise their products in the informational pamphlets, and there is some conflict with the aims of educating mothers about breastfeeding, but they do provide useful content that may help them [mothers]." She also mentioned that giving women a small present, such as a pamphlet, made them feel good about coming to see her and encouraged them to return for the additional sessions.

Session Two: The Video Presentation

Wang Yiqun, a twenty-four-year-old seamstress, enters the education room and announces that she is there for her second class on breastfeeding. Nurse Bai, who is busy talking to another woman, asks her to sit down next to me on the bench. As she is talking, she turns on the television and VCR, located to Wang Yiqun's right, and tells her to watch a video on breastfeeding. I watch the video with Wang Yiqun, as Nurse Bai continues to talk to the woman on the other side of the room. The video, titled *Muru Weiyang (Breastfeeding)* (Shanghai Educational Television 1994), opens with a picture of a chubby, healthy baby as the female narrator intones that breastfeeding is the most natural and scientific way to feed infants up to six months. The following description and summary of the video represents the elements that seemed most interesting to the women themselves.[9]

"Unfortunately, in the modern world, most people are not aware of the importance and benefits of breastfeeding," the narrator begins. This is followed by a montage sequence of workers in a laboratory examining what is presumably breast milk as the narrator outlines the more than one hundred beneficial substances contained in it. The film then cuts to a photograph of an infant's head, and an animated picture of the brain appears with the declaration that "these nutrients are essential for proper development of the brain." Viewers then see a smiling couple in a park with their infant, as the narrator reminds them that breastfeeding is also beneficial for mothers because it helps them to lose weight and avoid uterine problems during the postpartum period. Finally, as the camera moves in for a close-up of the smiling mother holding her infant, the narrator states that breastfeeding also encourages bonding and love between mother and child.

The next segment of the video takes us to an outpatient clinic where women are attending a breastfeeding class designed, according to the narrator, to help pregnant women better understand the "mysteries" of breastfeeding. The video then cuts to a diagram of the breast and describes the process of milk production and the relationship between nipple stimulation and the hormonal responses that encourage breast milk production. The filmed classroom shows women and their husbands—a situation that I never observed in the hospital where I conducted my research or in others that I visited. A medical professional in a white coat explains how milk is produced using a black and white line diagram. We then see a pregnant woman at home preparing her breasts for breastfeeding while the narrator states that the "work" of breastfeeding begins before birth. Women are told to toughen the nipples by rubbing them with a towel or washcloth at least thirty to forty times twice a day to avoid pain while breastfeeding.

The film describes birth briefly and without visual images. Instead, it focuses on a quick montage of women still in the delivery room with nurses helping them to breastfeed. These images then fade into a segment that demonstrates and discusses common problems women have when breastfeeding. Finally, we view a woman, returned home from the hospital with her infant while her husband brings a meal to the table with an abundant variety of dishes. The narrator tells us that the mother's nutrition during breastfeeding is important for milk production and the mother's health. The film continues with a depiction of a mother sleeping in a bed with her infant next to her (no husband) while we are told that "sleeping in the same bed with the infant is more convenient while breastfeeding and interferes less with the mother's sleep." The final sequence of images focuses on a group of young and old women admiring an infant as the narrator states, "Breastfeeding is an important means of improving the quality of the population (*renkou suzhi*) and future generations, and thus everyone shares a responsibility to promote it." "In the future," the narrator claims, breastfeeding "will be an important tradition for all mothers who raise healthy babies."

As noted earlier, I have excerpted those aspects of the video that seemed particularly interesting to the women in my study sample.[10] Other portions were included to illustrate the variety of messages conveyed to pregnant women in the breastfeeding class. We will look more closely at what these sessions conveyed to pregnant women below. For now let us turn to the final class attended by pregnant women in the Number 35 Hospital's obstetrics clinic.

Session Three: Learning How to Breastfeed

Zhang Yaoxin, a twenty-four-year-old secretary, at nine months is due to deliver in approximately two weeks. She sits down with a small groan, telling us that she is very uncomfortable—her feet and back hurt and she can't sleep through the night. Nurse Bai suggests that she soak her feet in warm water and try sleeping on top of an extra quilt to provide more cushioning for her back and sides. Nurse Bai asks Yaoxin to lift her shirt so she can check her nipples and breasts; she massages a breast and exclaims that it is well developed and her nipples are fine. She tells Yaoxin that she should have no problem breastfeeding and will have plenty of milk. She uses a plastic baby doll and a round cloth replica of a breast and nipple to show Yaoxin how to hold her baby to breastfeed. She then demonstrates how to remove the baby from the breast, explaining that an infant's sucking ability is very strong, and shows how to insert a finger at the side its mouth to break the suction before removing the baby from the breast. Yaoxin is given the doll and cloth for practice overseen by Nurse Bai, who tells her that after delivery her baby will be sleeping with her in the hospital room or ward. She tells Yaoxin that she might feel tired and uncomfortable in this situation, but the baby should breastfeed on demand and she must not use any bottles, water, juice, cow's milk, or milk powder as that might interfere with her own milk production.

Yaoxin nods and agrees with Nurse Bai throughout her lecture, and at the end she declares that she definitely plans to breastfeed because it is the natural (*zi ran*) way to feed an infant, to which Nurse Bai replies that she will raise a smart, healthy baby using her own milk. Nurse Bai also tells Yaoxin that she will be visiting her on the obstetrics ward after she gives birth to see if she has any questions or issues with breastfeeding. As Yaoxin gets up from the bench and moves to the door she replies, "Everything will be fine." These sessions relied on a variety of pedagogical means, from lectures to videos to practicing with model breasts and infants, in order to educate women about breastfeeding, and Nurse Bai seldom deviated from what has been presented here.

It is difficult, however, to describe any of the educational sessions I observed as routine for the women themselves. At times several women would be participating in the class, and often multiple conversations, examinations, and discussions occurred simultaneously. For the purposes of analysis here, however, these sessions provide a useful overview of the types of values, norms, and knowledge conveyed to women about their bodies and breastfeeding. For example, by noting that Zhang Yaoxin's enlarged breasts should provide plenty of milk, Nurse Bai communicated that enlarged breasts mean that good milk production will ensue. This is not necessarily the case for all women. Studies show that, in fact, some mothers will not produce breast milk as easily as others, and breast size seems to have little to do with production (Geddes 2007; Jelliffe and Jelliffe 1978). Zhang Yaoxin's expressions of discomfort with her pregnant body also prompted Nurse Bai to remind her that after birth she likely would continue to be uncomfortable but this should not deter her from breastfeeding. Nurse Bai, in her role as a medical expert, reinforced the idea that sacrifice is expected of mothers in the interest of their infants' well-being. Zhang Yaoxin, in her reactions to Nurse Bai, affirmed that she was willing to make sacrifices for her infant, especially as she shared the value of providing "natural" breast milk as opposed to "manufactured" infant formula. These moments of interaction, including Nurse Bai's lectures, monitoring of pregnant women's bodies through breast examinations, educational videos, and infant formula company pamphlets, demonstrate how health education, an essential component of the BFHI and a tactic in health promotion, can work to make clear the values and norms within which mothers may navigate on behalf of their infants (Foucault 1990; Bourdieu 1977; Gastaldo 1997.

The forces at work in shaping women's infant feeding decisions, however, were met with the women's responses to the mandatory classes, which echoed the conflation of science and nature found in the class sessions. Twenty of the thirty women in this study were resistant to the idea of having to attend the breastfeeding classes. They expressed their opposition in a variety of ways. Some voiced their resistance to me after class when I would meet with them. As Zhai Xiurong, a twenty-five-year-old factory manager, said to me one day, "Why should I have to attend a class? Breastfeeding and being a mother are natural; I don't need to go to a class to learn anything." When I asked her to whom she would turn if she needed advice, she told me, "My mother. She raised two children; she can help me." Zhai Xiurong's response was not an unusual one although more than half of the thirty women I followed told me that they would ask a doctor if they felt they had problems or questions during pregnancy. Other women resisted the class requirement by cutting the time spent in the session short, telling Nurse Bai they had an appointment or that their mother-in-law was waiting for them. Later, when I asked about the class sessions, some women stated that they simply did not want to stay and felt they did not need the information. Sun Limei, a thirty-year-old factory worker, was particularly reluctant to participate in the classes. When I met her afterward to talk, she told me that the classes were wasting her time.

> I do not believe that we should be required to attend this breastfeeding class. I do not need to have a nurse tell me how to do this. It is natural and normal to breastfeed. Why should I pay the hos-

> pital money to sit in a class that is useless? I cannot afford to waste time and money on such things. If I have a breastfeeding problem, then I can ask someone, but I do not have time for this class.

Other women who believed that the class was not necessary still attended and participated in discussions with Nurse Bai. Many of these women shared the view of Shen Jun, a twenty-four-year-old who worked in her husband's family's ice cream and novelty drink business.

> I come to these classes, but I am not certain they are really going to be very useful to me. Sometimes, though, you think that something like this is useless and later you might find out it was helpful, so I come. I am required to do this.

By contrast, seven women in my sample told me they enjoyed attending the class sessions. They felt that they needed information about breastfeeding and the classes addressed their concerns about raising a healthy child. Lu Bin, a twenty-seven-year-old manager in a publishing house, told me that she felt there were many aspects of child care that were more modern than the traditional ones used by her mother and mother-in-law. She did not want to raise her child using traditional and backward (*luohou de*) practices. She viewed the hospital staff in general and the breastfeeding class in particular as useful sources of modern knowledge and information about mothering.

> These classes are useful. I have learned many aspects of breastfeeding that are important. I want to raise a healthy, intelligent child, and I need to know the most scientific and advanced ways to do this. So I think classes like this are good for women like me who need to learn more about these issues.

Yan Daifeng, a printshop worker with a middle-school education, commented to me, "These classes are good because they help me think about how to best feed my infant, and I want to know what the best ways to raise children are—so these classes are good! Gu Lijian echoed Yan Daifeng's comments and also saw the classes as connecting her to the world: "I want the most scientific and up-to-date information to help feed my infant. This hospital, with its United Nations certification, is providing an international standard to us in these classes." These women and four others were also avid consumers of books on pregnancy and child care, and, as will become apparent in later chapters, they believed that knowledge obtained from authorities outside their families would help empower them as modern mothers. What we can conclude from all the women's comments and actions is that they managed the mandatory nature of these classes in ways that suited them and that this was an important instance when creative pragmatism became visible.

The Science and Nature of Motherhood

In the breastfeeding classes women encountered a biomedical model of pregnancy and infant feeding, the overarching authority of which rested in the use of science and nature to define these shared bodily experiences. Further, the universalizing character of these experiences reflects the rhetoric not only in formula company pamphlets but also in the information from UNICEF/WHO presented by Nurse Bai in her classes and videos. These materials assert that breastfeeding is a universal, biological function for women. The goal is then to seek ways to mitigate the limiting factors of "culture" and increase the rate of breastfeeding.[11] Earlier attempts to increase breastfeeding by the WHO and NGOs relied on the long-standing public health practice of discerning indigenous cultural practices that might inhibit breastfeeding initiation or supplementary feeding practices. Health workers then set out to persuade women to avoid such situations and change practices considered antithetical to breastfeeding.[12] This approach to changing health behavior makes the critical assumption that women's choices result from ignorance of healthier practices and once they know better they will change their behavior. With the advent of the BFHI in the early 1990s, however, the model of how to change health behavior adopted a more sophisticated approach, which acknowledged that increasing breastfeeding requires more than simply educating mothers about the benefits of breast over bottle.[13] That approach, as discussed in the "Introduction" and chapter 1, rests on the UNICEF/WHO assumption that the appeal of modernity is strongly associated with biomedicine and implementing breastfeeding programs in the hospital, a modern institution, could reinforce these connections and their cachet (United Nations 1996). However, we see in the breastfeeding classes this dual message in action: breastfeeding is both scientific and natural.

This logic also appears in the formula companies' informational pamphlets handed out by Nurse Bai, most of which also advertise their infant formula products. The WHO's Code on the Marketing of Infant Formula requires all formula company products and promotional materials to indicate that breastfeeding provides the best nutrition for infants up to the age of six months (World Health Organization 1981). The pamphlets distributed by Nurse Bai in the prenatal education classes all conform to this rule but vary in the content they present on breastfeeding. I analyzed twelve different pamphlets that I received from Nurse Bai and found that about half (seven out of twelve) present detailed information about the benefits and techniques of breastfeeding in both text and images. The others contain the brief message required by the WHO Cde while the remainder of the text addresses issues such as maternal nutrition, exercise, and the product line of the company. The twofold message in those pamphlets reiterates that breastfeeding is the most natural and scientific way to feed one's infant. One pamphlet contains a cover picture of a mother shaped like a pod with a tiny green sprout extending from her belly; inside the pamphlet, the infant is shown resting in a peapod-shaped plant. From the visual image alone, the message might be read that "growing" a baby is like nurturing a seed into a plant, and in the modern world that requires both nature and science. Akin to agricultural technology, then, infant formula works as a technology that relies on nature and science to produce a healthy infant. The message suggests that technology can help ensure that the potentiality and future of the infant can be managed. Usually the "science" of breastfeeding in these pamphlets is not expanded upon in the text. Instead, there is a statement that if for some reason a mother cannot use breast milk to feed her infant the company's infant formula product is a modern and scientific alternative. Pamphlets also often use charts and graphs, symbols of scientific information in themselves, to compare the formula's nutrients with those of breast milk and graphically demonstrate that the company's product is scientifically similar to breast milk. The play between nature and science is exemplified in one pamphlet in which large characters read, "The natural first choice for breast milk replacement" (*tidai muru de tianran shouxuan*). The message continues in smaller characters to note that breastfeeding is best for infants up to the age of six months, but for some breastfeeding is impossible and therefore this formula is naturally parents' first choice. Here formula is linked to nature by reversing language. Nature is not associated rhetorically with breastfeeding, as is usually the case, but rather with the manufactured infant formula. Ultimately, infant formula and breastfeeding are made equivalent in these advertisements for both are natural and scientific.[14]

The video that women watched in the breastfeeding class reinforced the dialectic of nature and medicine (or science). Pictures of laboratory workers making slides of breast milk and lists of the more than one hundred nutrients available in it, as well as the animated images of the hormonal/physiological aspects of milk production, are provided to convince the viewer of this dialectic. Medical authority in the form of interactions between health professionals and patients also appears throughout the video: images of nurses and doctors educating women and men about breastfeeding, nurses helping women learn correct positioning of the baby, nurses teaching women how to express breast milk, and nurses correcting mothers-in-laws who try to bottle-feed the baby by showing them the nutritional value of breast milk. The message is clear: breastfeeding, though natural, requires expert medical assistance. In a larger sense, the video conveys the idea that mothers require assistance in developing their mothering practices and medical knowledge, and thus medical authorities represent the best, most modern means through which to achieve this ideal. Most interesting is that the BFHI video and formula company pamphlets rely on the same intertwined ensemble of medical expertise, nature, science, and modernity as they seek to influence women's decisions to either breast- or bottle-feed their infants.

The twists and turns continue if we look at how nationalist futures and consumerist priorities are embedded in the representations and ideals conveyed to women during the breastfeeding class. It is in these priorities that we can see how nationalist interests in infant feeding intersect with women's interests in producing a healthy child. Several threads of rhetoric running through the formula company pamphlets, the educational video, and the class sessions are consistent with the one-child policy and the ideals of producing a strong citizenry for the future of China as a modern nation.[15] The formula pamphlets frequently linked children's intelligence to the use of their products. One pamphlet's graphic illustration does not require any facility with the Chinese language to understand the message; it consists of an outline of a child's brain containing many mathematical symbols. The implication is that if one uses the company's product the child will develop superior intelligence. Moreover, the use of mathematical symbols, a foundation of scientific reasoning, reinforces the association of the product with modernity. It is in such materials that we can see how state priorities become enmeshed in consumer products and offer yet another instance of the means of maternal governance asserting themselves in the hospital.

In the video, the final messages directly promote the nation's quest to improve the quality of the population and advise that breastfeeding is one important means of achieving this goal. For example, the video exhorts viewers to endorse breastfeeding as a part of their responsibility to society and the larger social good. The image accompanying this message shows a group of older women surrounding a younger woman holding an infant. These messages and representations thus link breastfeeding and motherhood to the future of the nation. It is women's individual and collective responsibility to produce superior, intelligent future citizens. Such lofty messages play into women's concerns about ensuring the health and intelligence of their only child; however, the women are also learning in their classes that breastfeeding is not the only means to such ends.

Nurse Bai brought infant formula into the classroom for pragmatic reasons. She handed out pamphlets advertising prenatal nutritional drinks produced by companies that also made infant formula; in her role as "breastfeeding educator," her medical authority lent weight to the claims made by the pamphlets. Giving women information supplied by infant formula companies during a breastfeeding class certainly contradicted the stated goals and practices of the BFHI. Nurse Bai, however, believed that in addition to her work to promote breastfeeding she had a responsibility to support women's health and well-being. While less than ideal given their association with infant formula, she found the information on maternal nutrition in the pamphlets useful for her patients. These actions resonate with Tine Gammeltoft's research (2014) on selective reproduction in Vietnam, where physicians, as cadres of the state, offer advice to women about whether to abort a fetus with anomalies but view this as a moral responsibility to the mother as much as the fulfillment of their duty to the state. These findings remind us that state power and the disciplinary forces found in policies do not simply function in a top-down manner. Rather, in the implementation of policies like the BFHI the interactions between nurses and pregnant women reflect qualities of caring and responsibility.[16] On another level, Nurse Bai's strategy, as well as justifications for it, represents another manifestation of the contradiction established in the assumption that breastfeeding is simultaneously natural and scientific. For, if breastfeeding is natural, why do women need to attend a class? Nurse Bai, by using the glossy pamphlets to provide information and serve as small gifts, implicitly acknowledged that an incentive might be necessary to encourage women to attend. Yet, if breastfeeding is also the most scientific and modern means of feeding infants, then the medical authority of science, combined with Chinese women's consumerist desires to achieve modernity in their self-representation, might in fact prove more powerful than any advertisement for infant formula. In sum, the BFHI's educational program for pregnant women draws on representations of breastfeeding as the embodiment of science, nature, and modernity to convince women to breastfeed. The contradictions and intersections of the science and nature of breastfeeding in the class sessions at the Number 35 Hospital, however, were made more meaningful, and indeed material, in the deeds of Nurse Bai. As she worked to educate her patients with the best materials at hand, Nurse Bai's actions in these classes can help us see that "the ways in which we know and represent the world are inseparable from the ways in which we choose to live in it (Jasanoff 2004, 4). In this instance, multiple ways of knowing and representing breastfeeding in the BFH introduced the possibility of bottle-feeding as an equally viable option through which to meet the goal of using the most scientific and modern means to nourish infants for the family and the nation.

Weighing Possibilities

Conflicting messages about the maternal body in relation to infant feeding and bodily self-presentation are threaded throughout Nurse Bai's classes, the breastfeeding education video, the formula company pamphlets, and the hallway posters. Specifically, one of the benefits of breastfeeding described by the video—over images of a slim, contented-looking woman strolling with her husband and baby in the park—is that breastfeeding promotes postpartum weight loss. Yet the video, at a later point, reminds women that they must eat more food while breastfeeding to ensure adequate nutrition for both the mother and her infant. It graphically represents the increase in calories needed by the mother's body to produce breast milk, while the narrator states that it is harmful to the mother and baby if the mother eats poorly or does not eat a wide variety of foods. One image in the video during this message shows a husband and wife sitting at a table in their apartment with an array of eight different dishes (Shanghai Educational Television 1994). When I asked the women in my study how many dishes they ate during an "average" dinner, most said they had two dishes with rice and sometimes three. Many women thought the food scene presented in the video was excessive and unrealistic. As Lu Bin put it, "The video shows the husband and wife eating enough food to feed eight people! No family eats like that every day." The clinic's hallway poster depicting lobsters and exhorting women to eat healthy foods, alongside the images of an unusually large meal depicted in the video, project rather unrealistic possibilities for consumption that these women clearly understand. Despite women's awareness of the idealized nature of these messages—that the consumption of such out-of-reach foods is connected to a healthy pregnancy or postpartum recovery—the message helps to create an environment in the hospital where the imperatives of good health and consumption are explicitly linked.

Health, consumption, and weight were also connected in women's concerns as they contemplated breastfeeding and weight gain during pregnancy. The pamphlets and video prompted much conversation about these issues among women in the study sample. During their pregnancies, most were not concerned about regaining their shapes; twenty-seven out of thirty women believed it would happen naturally without the need for exercise or dieting. Che Yan, the twenty-six-year-old woman who owned a small print-shop with her husband, described these pamphlets and images about body image as antithetical to pregnancy.

> If you want a healthy baby, of course you must gain weight. The fetus needs to be nourished, and your body must provide this. It is also growing, so of course you gain weight. But once you have given birth, your body will lose the weight from pregnancy. I do not worry about this now. After the birth I will lose the weight—most of it will be the infant!

Yang Huizhi, a twenty-three-year-old store clerk, reiterated Che Yan's outlook on this issue.

> It is natural during pregnancy to gain weight, and it is best for the baby's health if you gain weight. Some women worry about staying fat after the birth, but I think if you return to your normal eating you will lose the weight. The food in the video was too much! We never eat so many dishes whether I am pregnant or not.

However, ten women (one-third of my sample) told me that breastfeeding makes one gain weight, and they were concerned about this.

When I pointed out that the video they had watched claimed that breastfeeding contributed to weight loss, several women told me that this was not true based on what they knew about their friends' or relatives' experiences. One woman, Ke Hong, a twenty-six-year-old shop attendant, told me in her seventh month that she knew from the breastfeeding classes that it was best to breastfeed one's infant.

> I know that breastfeeding is the most nutritional way to feed an infant, but my sister had to eat a lot while she was breastfeeding, and she could not lose weight after she gave birth. She was always hungry. I think breastfeeding makes you hungry, and so you do not lose the weight from pregnancy. She has stopped breastfeeding, but she is still overweight and feels unattractive now. I will try to breastfeed and just not eat too much so that maybe I will not stay fat after my baby is born.

Wang Zhiyin, a factory worker, reflected on the video's message and what she had observed among her coworkers.

> It [the video] tells us that we must eat a lot to produce enough breast milk. It also tells us that breastfeeding will help us lose weight after giving birth. This is not what I have seen in the factory or my apartment building. Most women, if they breastfeed, seem to keep part of the weight from their pregnancies. My neighbor who had a child last year breastfed for three months, but she did not lose weight until she started using infant formula.

The variety of comments illustrates that women sought to balance apprehensions about their bodies with the well-being of their gestating infant. In spite of ten women voicing their belief that one could not lose weight while breastfeeding, all of these women, much as Ke Hong did, expressed interest in trying it first and seeing if it really presented a problem. Such perspectives help to illuminate that in the time frame of becoming a mother women anticipated the parameters and constraints they might face at later moments in the process of nourishing their infants.

Sexuality was never directly broached in the video or the pamphlets, but one sequence of scenes indicates that sleeping in the same bed with a husband while breastfeeding is incompatible with caring for an infant. As the narrator describes strategies for feeding on demand, the images shift to the bedroom where we see a woman with her newborn infant preparing for sleep. The husband is invisible, and the narrator suggests that mothers who sleep with their babies can conveniently breastfeed while remaining in bed and suffering fewer disruptions during the night. The final shot in the sequence shows a woman on a double bed with her infant sleeping next to her (Shanghai Educational Television 1994). Presumably the husband is sleeping on the couch! When I asked the pregnant women in my study what they thought about this message in the video, they all agreed that the infant should sleep with the mother. Several women suggested that if the bed were small, it would be best if the husband slept elsewhere at least for the first month. After the first month, when many women anticipated completing the ritual seclusion of "doing the month" (*zuo yuezi*; see chapter 4), they thought the baby could be moved to a crib or basket near the bed and that the husband should sleep with them. Beyond sleeping arrangements, the majority of women were not concerned with the timing or necessity of resuming sexual relations with their husbands during the prenatal portion of my research. Qu Wen, a twenty-five-year-old pharmacy technician in her fifth month, explained one day, "It is natural for mothers to sleep with their young children. When I was growing up in the countryside, we all slept together; no one thought about it."

However, five women talked about the fact that pregnancy and breastfeeding would interfere with their husband's sexual needs. These women expressed some concern that their husbands would seek sex with a prostitute. Some feared that their spouse might even fall in love with someone else while they were pregnant and breastfeeding. Cui Zhuhong, a twenty-seven-year-old office manager in her seventh month of pregnancy, met with me, and when I raised the issue of the video's content regarding sleeping arrangements she laughed and said, "I know what you are asking about. I worry that my husband has sexual needs now! I do not know if he can wait. I sometimes think that he might look for someone to go to bed with—I don't mean a prostitute, but there are women who are lonely." Once the women gave birth, their anxiety about sexual issues increased. Later chapters show that their feelings about juggling the competing demands on their bodies, time, and self-identity became more evident in their narratives.

Nurse Bai's concerns were different. In all the sessions I observed, she never mentioned the mother's body shape, weight, or sexual issues. She focused only on the psychological and physical benefits of breastfeeding for the infant and ways to maintain the mother's health. In fact, at one point I asked her if the training she had received at the UNICEF/WHO workshops ever raised issues of sexual relations. She responded that it never came up, and in her opinion it was an issue that was the business of individual women. Then she pulled out the training manuals she received at the workshop and told me to note that there was no information on sexual relations and breastfeeding. She did acknowledge that there were "traditional" beliefs about the appropriate time to resume sexual relations, and that for some people this meant waiting until after "the month" had been completed. Medically, she said, doctors in the hospital recommended that women wait at least until their six-week checkup before resuming sexual intercourse.

The representations of the reproductive female body in the spaces of the hospital, as illustrated in the breastfeeding video, the exercise pamphlets, and the hallway posters, ostensibly focus on health and well-being. Other layers of meaning in these media emphasize that the maternal body requires discipline and regimentation to ensure a return to a prepregnancy state-of-health and recovery of a body shape that erases its association with reproduction. Women's varied responses to these representations during pregnancy and the breastfeeding classes indicate that, within a constrained field of possibilities, they pragmatically assessed how to achieve a balance among a number of compelling and often competing demands on their bodies. These assessments, whether realized in actual practice, such as exercising or eating, or not, illuminate an important moment when the material body meets the idealized one. The seemingly practical information on breastfeeding and diet regimes presented in the classroom also shows that female bodies in urban China at that moment were "bodies whose forces and energies are habituated to external regulation, subjection, transformation, and 'improvement'" (Bordo 1993, 91).

Feminizing the Motherly Body

But women's narratives also show vividly that the body is not simply a blank slate on which multiple messages leave their mark. At every turn, new mothers construct, revise, or reaffirm aspects of their bodily sense of self amid the constellation of power relations that make up the world of the BFH. For instance, in its use of visual media to promote breastfeeding, the hospital environment also transmitted consumer values to women. The glossy poster of a sexually attractive breastfeeding mother in pearls and makeup (fig. 2) resonated closely with images of women found in other advertisements and promotions of consumer goods in Chinese magazines, television commercials, and billboards, to name a few.[17] Yet, in the hospital, these were juxtaposed with posters that contained such slogans as "Breastfeeding is best" (*muru weiyang shi zui hao de*), "help mothers achieve breastfeeding" (*bangzhu muqin shixian muru weiyang*), and "breastfeeding protects your precious one" (*muru baohu nide baobao*). The contrast between these messages was not lost on women when they visited the clinic. The image in figure 2 of the Asian woman in a glamorous negligee nursing her baby attracted spontaneous comments from several of them. One day as we walked down the clinic hallway, Wang Yiqun, the twenty-four-year-old seamstress, laughingly remarked, "That is a mistress (*xiaomi*) breastfeeding, not an ordinary mother." When Wang Yiqun described the breastfeeding mother in the poster as a mistress she was articulating her apprehension over the sexual message of the image. Her laughter and tone of incredulity indicated that breastfeeding and sexuality were incongruous at best in her mind. Indeed, as we continued our conversation after her comment, she told me that the image represented something out of reach for an ordinary woman like her. When I asked how she felt about that, she replied, "My husband would like it, but it is not me." Others noted the poster as well. One day, as we sat in the clinic hallway waiting for her checkup, Du Yan, a twenty-four-year-old woman in her fifth month of pregnancy, nodded toward the poster and asked in an ironic tone, "How can this beautiful woman also have time to breastfeed?" Finally, Lu Bin, the twenty-seven-year-old publications manager, commented when I asked her what she thought of the poster, "I like those pearls! You know you can buy them for a good price at the Pearl Market near Tiantan." These comments represent a variety of perspectives about the way the consumer body may or may not operate as a capital good in the eyes of different individuals (Ferry 2001). Du Yan, calling attention to the unrealistic portrayal of the breastfeeding mother, found the level of self-care and adornment incompatible with infant care. Lu Bin, by identifying the pearls as a commodity to which she has access, conveyed to me and herself that she could realize at least one aspect of the ideal portrayed in the poster. Despite differences in their responses, all three women were aware that the ideal body provides a means of achieving social prestige or opportunities through physical management, adornment, and presentation. Certainly, the image conveys the message that women can, if they adopt the poster woman's style, dress, and comportment, add the sexually attractive, breastfeeding mother to their self-identity. But their comments also suggest that it is possible to critique, reject, or only partially accept the possibilities imbued in the image.[18] These brief remarks also show that the multiplicity of responses to bodily management and its potential contribution to women's social capital continue to matter during pregnancy.

Portable Pressures: Exercising the Maternal Body

While breastfeeding posters formed a fixed aspect of the hospital environment, the formula company pamphlets distributed by Nurse Bai during the breastfeeding classes were portable and could be read in more detail by the women. These texts use scientific images and medical language to justify the achievement of a healthy body during pregnancy (presumably assisted by use of their product). Yet they, too, had the potential to reinforce women's worries about beauty and attractiveness. For example, a pamphlet produced for Mead Johnson's maternal supplement powder drink, MaMa Sustagen (rendered in English in the pamphlet), includes a series of exercises for the prenatal and postpartum periods featuring a slim, leotard-clad woman. The information provided in the text outlines the importance of maternal nutrition for the healthy development of the fetus. The photographic images of a woman performing exercises and the accompanying text tell the reader that performing the postnatal exercises, mostly sit-ups, will help a woman return to her prepregnancy shape, heal the perineal area, and prevent prolapse of the uterus.[19] The message is clear: the feminine body, not the pregnant one, must be restored as soon as possible after birth. The glossy, slim woman in the pamphlet photo sequence is certainly not pregnant, nor does she look like most women in the immediate postpartum period. Presuming that her body is meant to represent the postpartum woman, it differs dramatically from the bodies of pregnant or newly delivered women, who are inevitably living with a larger body. Ultimately, the pamphlet places an additional demand on new mothers so that along with a safe birth and a healthy infant, it is now desirable to have a body that quickly returns to a prepregnancy state of slimness.

And if a reader doesn't find this particular message compelling, the pamphlet introduces new types of health risks and concerns to the reproductive process in the form of uterine prolapse. The presentation of these exercises as a remedy for such postpartum complications can be read, on the one hand, as introducing new types of medical risks women may face during their recovery from birth. However, they also might be read as markers of the success of the Chinese state in improving maternal and child survival since 1949, for the pamphlet's producers assume that most women will survive childbirth and recover—something that could not be taken for granted in earlier times. The pamphlet's message conveys these dual meanings and at the same time represents the public health promotions of the mid-1990s, which emphasized that achieving good health through the actions and behavior of individuals, rather than institutions, will minimize the risk of illness, or in this case uterine prolapse.[20]

The messages advocating exercise during pregnancy, however, did not seem to strongly influence the women in this study. Of the thirty women I followed, only five exercised in either their pre- or immediately postnatal periods. In fact, when I asked these women what they thought about the exercises described in the pamphlets, many of them laughed. Several said, "I have no time; it is not for me," or, as Han Aihua stated, "If I had a body like that, I wouldn't have to exercise." Yan Daifeng, the printshop worker, told me that she got plenty of exercise bicycling to work a half hour each way and doing her job. But she noted, "I do a lot of lifting and carrying of heavy boxes of papers—this has made me strong. But now that I am pregnant, I do not lift anything very heavy, and soon I will be leaving my job because it is too strenuous for me while I am pregnant. If I sit at a desk all day, I will get even fatter."

As I examined these pamphlets with the women in my study, I found that their reactions to the idea of exercise during pregnancy were fairly uniform: it was not necessary. Xie Jinmei, a twenty-four-year-old woman who originally came from a village on the outskirts of Beijing, explained that women's work at home and in the workplace provided exercise enough: "My job in an electronics factory is hard work. I carry boxes, stand or walk all day, and ride my bicycle to work. I also shop for food almost every day, and we live on the fifth floor of an apartment building! I get more than enough exercise every day; these exercises [depicted in the pamphlet] may be suitable for women who don't have much to do either at home or at work. If you are healthy and able to participate in daily life, exercise during pregnancy is not important." Despite the fact that the majority of the women did not engage in formal exercise, this did not reflect a lack of concern for their physical shape.

Most women raised issues of their changing body shape, weight, and muscle tone at various times during their pregnancies. Yang Huzhi, a young department store worker her sixth month of pregnancy, began our conversation one day with an exclamation: "Look at my belly! I have grown so big, and my body is changing. I just keep getting bigger and bigger!" She pulled up her shirt to show me that she was wearing a pair of men's pants several sizes too large for her and held up with a belt, "Look! I am wearing my husband's pants because nothing I have will fit me. I know I will lose weight after the baby comes, but look at me!" Though expressing concern with the bodily changes she was experiencing, Yang Huzhi remained confident that she would lose weight after childbirth. She was not necessarily expressing anxiety about her body in our conversation but more a sense of wonderment and a bit of exasperation at having to wear her husband's pants. Zhou Xiuying, a thirty-year-old nurse at the Number 35, said in her sixth month that because of her enlarged breasts she had to buy new bras and shirts.

> Last Saturday I went to the department store to buy new bras and shirts with my husband. He was joking with me about my bigger breasts and wondered if my friends and coworkers would think I had had plastic surgery as I have not developed such a large belly; many people might not notice that I am pregnant. But they are not that big! I have gained weight, but it is not showing in my stomach. My mother told me that her pregnancies were like this. The good thing is that she told me that once she gave birth, her belly shrank pretty quickly. I hope that I am the same way.

Her husband's joke about Xiuying's larger breasts being attributed to breast enhancement surgery rather than pregnancy reflects the relatively new and rapidly developing availability of plastic surgery as a way to correct or enhance body parts. In the mid-1990s, women's magazines contained stories and advertisements about plastic surgery as a solution to numerous beauty "problems" ranging from reshaping eyelids and noses to breast enhancement, but they were characterized as relatively extreme solutions because they were costly and not widely available to the average person. In the years since this study, however, plastic surgery seems to have gone mainstream. A Chinese friend in 2005 told me about a beauty pageant for women who had undergone plastic surgery that received national attention when one contestant was turned away for having had too many procedures, making it impossible for others to compete with her. Such a celebration of surgically induced beauty and physical perfection suggests that in China the social and cultural link between bodies and prestige has continued to intensify in the twenty-first century (Luo 2013). As much as the joke about breast size captures our attention, however, Zhou Xiuying also spent a good part of our discussion describing and analyzing her weight gain and anticipating a speedy recovery to her prepregnancy size, thus indicating her confidence at this moment that her body would conform to expectations such as those exhibited in the pamphlet.

Confidence in a rapid recovery of the prepregnancy body was not shared by a few of the women. Feng Dongxin, a thirty-three-year-old administrator in her fourth month, expressed concern that she did not have time to exercise and that her age would make it more difficult to regain her prepregnancy shape.

> I do not exercise because I don't have time. I am still working, and when I come home I still have to do many household chores. My husband helps me, but he works too. So I don't exercise. Sometimes I think that since I am older, I should take better care of myself. I have not gained a lot of weight yet, but I know that it is difficult when you get older to lose weight. I think that maybe after I have the baby, I will have time to exercise more. My mother will come and live with us after the birth, and I will have a leave from my job. Maybe then I can exercise more and lose the weight I will gain from this pregnancy.

Like Feng Dongxin, most of the thirty women said that work and household duties did not permit the indulgence of special exercises. That most women described their daily lives and the physical demands made on their bodies as strenuous during pregnancy also reflects the fact that, at least in this study sample at this time in Beijing, there were no significant differences in lifestyle between white-collar women and factory or small business women. These women were all subject to similar physical demands in terms of commuting on bicycles or buses, almost daily food shopping, and household chores. Such similarities suggest that significant material differences in daily life had yet to manifest themselves among these groups.[21] I didn't find, for example, that women in white-collar jobs had easier daily lives than women in factory jobs.

A stated awareness of the physical demands of their daily lives seemed to shape most women's belief that special exercise was not necessary. A thread that also connected these women's responses was that of time. The timing of my questions about exercise occurred during pregnancy when these women, having never experienced this process, were optimistic about many aspects of their future lives as mothers. Their bodies, they expected, would quickly recover from pregnancy and childbirth. They thus envisioned a bodily future based not on experience but on identification with the projected norms surrounding them in the hallways of the hospital, in popular media, and in the experiences of female kin or friends, to name a few. The prominence of time as a measure of age, though only expressed directly by one of the older women in this study, also underlies the women's lack of interest in formal exercise programs. That Feng Dongxin worried that her age would inhibit her ability to recover her prenatal body while the younger women seemed buoyed with confidence that they would lose their pregnancy weight without much effort can be seen to reflect assumptions about the resilience of youthful bodies. Yet the pamphlets convey a different message: whether old or young, pre- and postnatal women's bodies require control. The onus for managing these bodies rests on women's ability to exert self-control through exercise to prevent medical conditions and speed recovery of the prepregnancy body. According to this message, the mother's body does not naturally recover from childbirth but requires intervention based on expert advice. Science, with its exercise regime, the pamphlet suggests, can both remedy the potential medical consequences of childbirth and promote women's consumerist desire for a slim body. In chapters 4 and 5, women's responses to this form of authority are taken up in more detail.

Conclusion

The constellation of relations embedded in the hospital environment conveyed a multidimensional field of potentiality in the images and ideals of motherhood, infant feeding, and the feminine body. Throughout the breastfeeding education process and the physical spaces of the obstetrics clinic, these potentials were expressed to and experienced in multiple ways by women. Underlying the rhetoric of this trio of representations rests the binary logic of nature and culture, the weight of medical authority, and consumerism. Women navigated these dynamics in different ways. Some, on the one hand, believed that they had no use for a breastfeeding class but on the other still found the pamphlets' promotion of femininity through exercise regimes a positive benefit. Interestingly, women's reactions to the classes did not correlate with their occupations or educational backgrounds and indicated the difficulty of locating commonalities in the ways individuals respond to health education. Indeed, in this instance, the interactions created in the breastfeeding classes and the meanings given to them by the pregnant women and Nurse Bai worked to coproduce multiple meanings and ways of responding to the BFHI.

The following chapters continue to show the ways in which consumerism, medical authority, and the nature/culture framework asserted themselves and were received as these pregnant women became mothers and made decisions about feeding their infants.

In the intervening years, the presence of infant formula advertising and products in hospitals and stores has increased dramatically, and researchers have documented flagrant violations of the WHO Code and China's laws prohibiting the promotion and distribution of infant formula in hospitals. A recent survey of mothers in six cities in China found that hospitals were providing free samples to 40 percent of the women in the study. The researchers also found that 60 percent of labels of infant formula did not contain the mandatory WHO Code statement that breastfeeding is the best way to feed an infant (A. Liu et al. 2014). China Central Television reported in 2013 that infant formula companies paid bribes to hospitals and health workers to recommend their formulas to new mothers (Zhao, Peng, and Yang 2014). Another news report from Qingdao found that free samples of infant formula were being distributed in hospitals that had been certified as baby friendly.[22] The constellations of relations that shape China's BFHs in the twenty-first century continue to reflect the contradictory and blurry dynamics found in the Number 35 Hospital, where women sought to determine the best way to feed their infants.

CHAPTER THREE

Anticipating Motherhood

Introduction

To anticipate birth in a hospital in China, or indeed anywhere, is to participate in a modern form of reproduction. Biomedical practices like those at the prenatal clinic of the Number 35 Hospital are often viewed as forces that define pregnancy as a medical problem under the guise of science and modernity.[1] The experience of and responses to this time among the women in this sample indicate that, despite receiving care in a hospital, most did not actively engage with the medical or biological dimensions of their pregnancies. In fact they assumed that others in positions of authority and knowledge, such as physicians and nurses, would oversee and anticipate their health care.[2] Anticipating motherhood, then, took on a double meaning. During pregnancy, women were simply looking forward to getting through the birth of their children. They also relied on female kin and friends, in addition to medical professionals, to anticipate their needs and ensure a healthy pregnancy and ultimately a healthy child. Most women did not avidly read the two popular books on pregnancy that were readily available in the hospital lobby. What initially looked to an outsider like a nonreactive stance toward the significant physical, personal, and social transformation that accompanies pregnancy requires reconsideration about the ways individuals shape their worlds and experiences. This chapter looks at the ways women navigated pregnancy, their changing bodies, their social relations, and their self-identity from the middle to the end of their pregnancies as they made plans to feed their infants. I look at this moment as one in which women traversed a range of imperatives derived from global and state policies, medical knowledge and practices, and their kin. In doing so, their intentions to breastfeed may reflect more than the success of the BFHI.

The breastfeeding classes described in chapter 2 provided a well-defined venue in which to highlight the ways in which health education translates a variety of forms of power into the microlevel practices and spaces of the hospital and what these can tell us about infant feeding and becoming a mother. Indeed, the classes aimed not only to increase women's understanding of the benefits of breastfeeding but also ultimately to influence their intention to breastfeed. Studies have found a strong association between women's intentions to breastfeed during pregnancy and their subsequent decisions to initiate and continue breastfeeding.[3] Research on pregnant women's intentions to breastfeed, in turn, focuses on social and demographic characteristics, such as maternal age, first pregnancy, care by midwives, and types of hospital, that correlate with women's plans to breastfeed or not. Yet, as the chapter will show, more than breastfeeding classes or demographics were at work in shaping how women anticipated the best ways to nourish their newborns.

I draw on the analytical framework of coproduction as a way to better represent and understand the dynamic nature of this moment. Typically, coproduction makes visible the ways in which scientific knowledge is produced and reproduced in a given context by key stakeholders who are products of particular cultural, political, and historical contexts.[4] In this case, while the BFH's promotion of breastfeeding operated as a centralized space in which to facilitate coproduction, other aspects of the prenatal care process within and outside the hospital walls also shaped ideas and practices about pregnancy, infant feeding, and mothering a healthy, intelligent child.

The first section of this chapter looks at the meanings of pregnancy, becoming a mother, and infant feeding from the perspectives of the women themselves and from a sample of popular pregnancy manuals. Following this discussion, we look at clinical encounters during prenatal visits and how women experienced and interpreted them and find that the women assumed that experts—physicians and nurses—would anticipate their health care needs. Outside the hospital, women relied on experienced female kin and friends to manage and understand the daily aspects of pregnancy. The web of relations on which they depended during their pregnancies both within and outside the hospital also helped to shape the range of possibilities for nurturing their infants. From the realm of physicians, family, and friends, this chapter then expands its scope to explore the ways in which "fetal education" connects China's traditions, state interests, and consumer culture with how women in the mid-1990s thought about these dynamics in their lives. In this way, we can see how coproduction might be applied to other epistemologies or systems of knowledge outside that of biomedicine. The chapter closes by showing that mid-1990s pregnancy advice books foreshadowed changes in the structures of authority, kin relations, institutions, care during pregnancy, and infant feeding practices in the twenty-first century. It is important to note that twenty-nine of the thirty women in this study intended, while in the hospital environment, to breastfeed. This link between the institution and individual women's decisions suggests the importance of state policies—the one-child policy and the BFHI—along with the patriarchal and patrilineal family system, and resulted in a situation that did not require their active participation in anticipating how to best nurture their infants.

Meanings of Pregnancy and Motherhood

During field research for this study, which began when the women in the sample were between four and six months pregnant, a perplexing situation developed. Given my prior experiences in the United States researching childbirth and infant feeding practices, I expected that women in this study would have a great deal to say about their pregnancies, their bodily experiences, and the meanings the whole process held for them. They did not. For example, there were no conversations about reaching the week in their pregnancy when the fetus developed the ability to hear or the moment when they first felt the fetus move, often referred to as quickening. My anticipation was not completely guided by my bias as a westerner. I had collected a number of popular manuals on pregnancy and infant feeding in Beijing and Harbin since 1991. At the time I began my research, I had already purchased 18 such books from local newsstands and bookstores in the area around the Number 35 Hospital. To date I have bought more than 200 of such books.[5] I assumed that, given the large numbers of books dealing with pregnancy, Chinese women must be participating or at least actively interested in the details of theirs. This assumption was somewhat misguided. When I asked women if they had purchased any of the popular manuals on the market, 28 out of 30 had done so at some point early in their pregnancies. However, when I asked if they had read or used them for information about their pregnancies, 23 women told me that they had not read them completely but used them as a reference, although 18 searched for information about birth as they approached their due dates.

During the first two months of meeting with the women in the study sample, I believed that the general reticence I encountered when asking about their pregnancies and bodily experiences was due to the circumstances: we were strangers, and this was an intimate topic. I was a foreigner, and moreover, I was childless. These factors certainly played a role in many of my early interviews, but as I came to know each woman, I found that generally they were not interested in discussing the nuanced aspects of their pregnancies. What did we discuss? Often we talked about their concerns with trying to work and be a good mother, whether the reforms had made women's economic situation better or worse, how American women give birth with the assistance of drugs, and how they were coping, in a daily sense, with being pregnant. It was only much later that I came to realize that their comments and discussions about their daily lives during pregnancy provided me, as an outsider, with a better understanding of their priorities. This is not to say that individual women did not feel the bodily changes of pregnancy and note them at times in our conversations, and I am certain they also did so with others. However, the details of the pregnancy did not emerge as a significant topic in these discussions.

Only after some time spent puzzling this out did I come to realize to what extent the social relations of caring entered into the majority of these women's narratives. What may look like passivity on the part of these women may be better viewed as their understanding that others, such as doctors, nurses, mothers, mothers-in-law, and husbands, would anticipate those situations during pregnancy requiring interventions, instructions, or knowledge. In the case of becoming a mother, these women considered pregnancy and childbirth to be times that require the assistance of persons with more expertise. Only after the child arrived did each woman become the caregiver of her infant.[6] That most women did not anticipate or concern themselves with the details of their pregnancies also reflected a belief in and reliance on the expert knowledge of medical professionals or the experiences of their female kin and friends. Underlying this approach was the belief that childbearing is a natural, not pathological, condition that requires women's active participation but only in ways that are within their control, such as eating properly and attending prenatal checkups at the hospital.

The women's social relations and expectations during pregnancy did not obscure their overall feelings about having a child. For the most part, they fell into three categories regarding their feelings about pregnancy and children: those that believed the process was a natural one not requiring much intervention, those that believed science and medicine were important to their pregnancies and the future health of their infants, and finally a small group of women (three out of thirty) that were seemingly indifferent to their pregnancies and the idea of having a child. Among those women who believed that pregnancy is a natural event that does not require much intervention, particularly medical intervention, there was some similarity in that for the most part their mothers grew up in rural China. Specifically, of the eleven women whose mothers came from rural areas, nine formed part of the group that viewed pregnancy as natural. Three women with urban backgrounds also believed that pregnancy does not require much intervention. Du Yan, a twenty-four-year-old buyer for a state factory whose mother came from rural Hebei Province, described the way she viewed reproduction.

> Pregnancy and childbirth are natural. I don't really think too much about all the things that the doctors and nurses tell me. I know that I need to eat food that is nutritious and maintain my health, but there is not much else that I need to worry about.

Among those women who expressed the belief that medicine and science are important to the reproductive process, most had mothers who grew up in urban areas. Of the nineteen women who had mothers of urban origin, thirteen described to me their concerns that pregnancy and childbirth required medical intervention. Furthermore, they frequently linked medicine to the health of their future children. Shi Binyan, a thirty-one-year-old engineer, made this connection in her comments to me during an interview in her eighth month of pregnancy.

> I want to have a healthy child. I am older and have had two miscarriages since I have been married. I think that doctors are the most important source of information during pregnancy. If I have a question, I ask them. They know what is best to protect me and the fetus.

This comment highlights the notion that women and their fetuses require protection during pregnancy and that physicians are most qualified to provide it. This may well be because Shi Binyan suffered two miscarriages before carrying the third pregnancy to term and thus felt particularly vulnerable. Her views may also reflect the fact that she is relatively well educated in a discipline associated with science. However, the pattern in my study sample is not so clear-cut. Wu Qiuping, a young factory worker with a middle school education also expressed her belief that medical intervention was necessary for her pregnancy and the well-being of her future child.

> I think that pregnancy and childbirth require western medicine. Since I can only have one child, I want it to be healthy and strong. Western medicine helps women protect their health, and this helps the fetus grow into a healthy infant.

Her words make clear that she views western medical intervention as a way to ensure the health of this only child. Others echoed Qiuping's sentiments. Bi Hongxia, a worker in her husband's family business, and Yang Huzhi, a store clerk, were sitting with me in the breastfeeding classroom one day, and the issue of medical intervention during childbirth came up in our discussion.

BI HONGXIA: My mother had a cesarean section when I was born. She recently told me that the placenta was located in such a way that if she tried to deliver normally she might die. She was lucky to be in a hospital when they discovered the problem. As I get closer to delivery, my mother has begun to tell me more about her experiences with childbirth.

YANG HUIZHI: My mother, too, has been telling me how fortunate I am to be able to see a doctor or midwife when I come to the hospital! I even get to visit the hospital before I give birth. She keeps telling me that when she had her first child in the countryside, she gave birth with an older neighbor to help. Her own mother was visiting relatives and could not get home. She is always telling me that I have nothing to worry about since I will have doctors and nurses to take care of me.

BI HONGXIA: I know! My mother-in-law's attitude is that I have nothing to worry about because I am able to receive medical care in a hospital. She says to me over and over, "This is your precious one, and you only get one, so you need to make sure you listen to the doctor and take care of yourself." I know she wants a healthy grandchild to carry on the family line. I think because she had difficulty getting pregnant and had one son die in a work accident she is more concerned than my own mother about this child. I am glad to be able to have modern medicine to help me and the fetus if necessary. I think I would worry a lot more.

YANG HUIZHI: Oh, me too! I know that this is natural, but I feel it is safer and better to be able to have the advice and examinations of doctors and nurses.

BI HONGXIA: Of course it is safer. Western medicine can help if there is an emergency; even if you do not need surgery, there are medicines and scientific technology to help. But I think Chinese medicine (Zhongyi) is helpful for complicated illness that is not easily cured in a short time. It can also help strengthen the body when it needs it. My mother makes me drink Chinese medical tonics everyday just to keep my body healthy.

These women are reminded that they have the responsibility to ensure the well-being of their future only child, but their primary responsibility, as expressed here, is to follow the advice of medical experts. The discussion between these women also demonstrates that older female kin, in recounting their own experiences of pregnancy and particularly childbirth in earlier times, transmit the value of receiving hospital-based medical care. It is such details, whether it is complications requiring a cesarean section or having to give birth attended by a nonrelative in a home setting, that convey the belief that risks can be minimized with medical expertise and support. Despite their agreement that pregnancy and childbirth are natural, as opposed to pathological, processes, the women's discussion emphasizes that risk is also present, and they accept that medical intervention may be required. Indeed, there is an element underlying their comments that suggests one has little control over these events, especially childbirth. Through a US cultural lens these women's responses might be read as unequivocal acceptance of the idea that pregnancy and childbirth require medical supervision and intervention. However, Ivry's research on pregnancy in Israel and Japan finds that during pregnancy Japanese women keep meticulous diaries of their bodily sensations, as well as those of the fetus's development, along with information from prenatal exams and ultrasound images (2009). These actions make legible a social script that emphasizes that pregnancy is a period requiring the mother's care for the fetus and a time of prenatal bonding between mother and fetus (180). By contrast, in Israel

Ivry finds what she calls the "trivialization of pregnancy"—because it is viewed as so commonplace. Interestingly, some pregnant women "ideologically cooperate in the trivialization of their own pregnancies" (188). They don't expect nor desire special treatment because they are pregnant. In 1990s China, women were not trivializing their pregnancies, nor were they documenting their bodily sensations and fetal development as ways to bond with their future children. Yet, as their conversation makes clear, individual responsibility for maintaining a healthy pregnancy is recognized as valuable and important to the women in this study. Others implement the actual practices, whether it is a mother who provides a Chinese herbal tonic to ensure her daughter's continued good health throughout her pregnancy or an admonition to follow doctor's orders.[7] With their understandings of the risks of pregnancy and childbirth, these women placed the potential and future outcomes in the hands of experts and experienced female kin.

Three women in the study sample seemed particularly uninterested in becoming mothers, and at times I found them rather reticent in our meetings, either at the hospital or in a nearby café. Two women were ambivalent about having a child but eventually, after giving birth, became interested in mothering. One woman, Gu Lijian, an administrator in a municipal construction office, was very clear that she was having the child in order to fulfill her duties to her husband's family.

> I do not really want to have a child, but it is my duty, so I am having it. But I do not want to raise it. My mother-in-law will take care of the baby. My husband also wants this child, so I told him I would have it but I do not want the responsibility of taking care of it.

Gu Lijian's reasons for not wanting a child and her reasons for having one are clearly linked to concepts of filial responsibility to one's in-laws and the expectation (one she reluctantly shared) that one should reproduce to continue the husband's family line. Though a rather dramatic departure from the other women's feelings about their impending motherhood, Gu Lijian's prenatal negotiations of her maternal role represent the success of the Chinese state's attempts to empower and liberate women from the Confucian family structure through participation in the labor force. In a later conversation, Lijian explained:

> I have a very busy job that I like. I am a manager for a construction company, and it is an exciting time to be working in this field. My work unit started this company as a specialized branch, and I was chosen to work there—it is a real honor, and I make a much better salary than before. I have never felt like I wanted children, maybe it was the way I was raised, but I just don't have the maternal instinct!

When I asked her how she reached the agreement with her mother-in-law, she replied:

> It was not easy. It took some time for her to realize that I was not trying to get permission to get pregnant, but once she did she put constant pressure on me. She would say things like "I want grandchildren; what will happen to our family if there is no new generation?" Or she would make comments when we saw an older woman with a child such as "Oh how I want to hold my grandchild, please give me a grandchild!" At first I tried to explain why I did not want a child, but eventually I just stopped responding to her. Then she put pressure on her son, my husband. My husband and I had never really talked about not having a child, but he understood that my work is important to me. But once she started on him, they both tried to convince me of my duty to the family, the future of our family, etc. I eventually agreed to have a child but only under my conditions—I did not want to be primarily responsible for raising it.
>
> SG: Why did they agree to this condition?
>
> Because I make a high salary and provide the most financial support to the family. I make their lives easier; I can afford to send my in-laws to travel—they visited Emei Mountain last year. My salary

> helped to renovate their apartment. I made sure my mother-in-law had a new kitchen with the most modern equipment since she does all the cooking. So now I have some power [with which] to come to an understanding with my family!

Lijian's description of her power to provide her family with a better life full of consumer goods and travel and her mother-in-law's lamentations about a grandchild represent one of the many quandaries that Chinese families faced in the mid-1990s. Gates's research among female small business owners in Chengdu and Taibei in the 1980s reinforces the notion that these questions and concerns about whether and how to have a child while continuing to work and find fulfillment in nonmaternal pursuits are long-standing (1995). Erwin also found in her research on Shanghai advice hotlines that the increasing affluence of urban families and the decline of state social welfare structures resulted in renewed privatization of social relationships and support within the family and that with these changes came new opportunities and challenges for women like Lijian (2000, 168–69).[8] As the following sections make clear, family support has helped to shape ideas about marital relationships, medical authority, and mothering. Finally, as the above discussion indicates, while all thirty women participated in the culturally and socially valued process of reproduction by becoming pregnant and eventually giving birth, their views about why they did so varied. This instance reinforces Cohen's suggestion that "common forms do not generate common meanings" (1994, 20). These variations remind us that the forms of maternal governance of the mid-1990s, whether prenatal checks, the actions of mothers and mothers-in-law, or popular pregnancy advice books, provided space for different responses from women.

Pregnancy by the Book

On the second day of my research at the Number 35, Dr. Zheng, the obstetrics department director, pointed out a small bookstand in the lobby where patients could find a variety of books on health. She told me that the bookstand was one attempt by the Number 35 Hospital to introduce revenue-producing schemes as the central government was beginning to require all hospitals to become more financially self-sufficient. At the same time, the selling of books on pregnancy, among other subjects, brought an element of China's expanding consumer culture into the immediate environment of the BFH. Furthermore, the sanctioning of the sale of particular pregnancy books in the hospital can be seen as reinforcement of their legitimacy for those who purchased them. And twenty-eight out of thirty women in this study bought at least one of two books on pregnancy at the hospital's bookstand on the recommendation of obstetrics clinic physicians. *Huai yun qian hou hua you sheng (Before and After Pregnancy: Remarks on Good Nurturing) (hereafter Before and After Pregnancy)* was most popular among the group and purchased by 26 women. Most women used them as a reference tool rather than an instruction manual on how to manage their pregnancies. The pregnancy books represent a form of consumption that brought socially and politically sanctioned ideas of how women should comport themselves during pregnancy into the hands of individuals seeking to negotiate the bodily and social changes that accompany becoming a mother.

I introduce aspects of the books as a way to connect these texts to the experiences that women discussed with me in our meetings. This connection is not merely rhetorical. As Farquhar shows in her work on bodies and embodiment in eating, sexuality, and medicine in post reform China (2002), texts have the power to produce embodied experiences. The books and women's pregnant bodies are products of a particular time and resonate with the social milieu of the present alongside visions of the past and future. Moreover, pregnant women's reflections about their bodies and the pregnancy books come to exist in the social realm through language (8). The buying and reading of such books or other media by women is an apt example of de Certeau's suggestion that consumption is a form of production. The production brought about by consumption, he argues, is created in the ways a product is used by the consumer, not in the creation of a new product (1984, xiii). Thus the purchase and reading of pregnancy books are not merely an act of consumption through the intake of information or ideas presented in the book. Rather, buying and reading such texts offer opportunities to use them in creative ways for women's own ends. The books are a single example of this process of consumption as production. Indeed, women experienced their pregnant bodies and consumed information from multiple sources within and outside the hospital, including media, family, friends, and medical professionals. The bodily transformations brought about by pregnancy not only required that all women acknowledge and articulate responses to such physical changes but also compelled them to continually negotiate the structures of medical knowledge, femininity, social support, and political agendas as imminent mothers.

In both books, care is expected to be provided by two individuals: the husband and the physician. For example, *Before and After Pregnancy* identifies the husband as a key support person in his pregnant wife's daily life (Li and An 1991). While two books were purchased by women in this study, *Before and After Pregnancy* was purchased by 28 out of 30 women. Line drawings in the book graphically illustrate appropriate ways for a husband to behave. For example, we see a man encouraging his pregnant wife on a walk outside, sitting and talking with his wife (the caption reads "Frequently have heart to heart talks"), and listening to music and singing to the pregnant woman. Finally, in the fourth drawing, a man is depicted with an apron around his waist bending over a stove with a caption that reads, "Do more of the household work" (40). The text also states, "After the wife is pregnant, more often than not the husband feels that the fetus no longer has anything to do with him; this is not the case" (40). To paraphrase the remainder of the section, it is suggested that the husband can protect the health of his future child by not smoking or drinking alcohol while his wife is pregnant. The authors also point out that the mother's psychological state is equally important to the development of the fetus. To this end, they exhort the husband, "After your wife is pregnant, the psychological anxieties as a result of the yearning for the child, reactions to unsuitable worries, dread of childbirth, [and] recovery from childbirth, these not only influence the pregnant woman herself but also can have a negative influence on the fetus" (40). Concerns about how women's psychological state, as they anticipate childbirth and the postpartum recovery, may affect the fetus's well-being may not seem particularly new to many readers. However, the suggestion that men might protect the health of the mother and fetus by not smoking and drinking extends their role beyond that of a caretaker to one of a participant. Moreover, such instructions, from the future father's behavior to the future mother's psychological well-being, raise the specter of potential problems that extend beyond the woman's pregnant body.

The weight placed on the role of the husband as protector, not only of his wife's physical condition but that of his future child, raises some interesting issues about potentiality and the social and cultural importance of caring for the pregnant woman. First, it suggests that pregnant women require specific types of physical, as well as psychological, support during this time if they are to produce a healthy child. In this case, the husband is identified as the individual who should take responsibility for his wife's well-being. For US readers, this advice may not seem unusual or strange. But in China, traditionally, the welfare of pregnant women has fallen to mothers and mothers-in-law rather than husbands. The images and advice presented in this manual are directed to a modern, nuclear family and emphasizes the marital bond as the central caring relationship during pregnancy. The women in my study did not often mention their husbands as their main source of support during pregnancy.[9] Almost all noted that their mothers-in-law, mothers, friends, sisters, or other female relatives were the key source of knowledge and social support.[10] This is not to say that husbands were completely absent. Many of the women related that their husbands were doing more household chores such as cleaning, cooking, and shopping. However, twenty-one of the thirty women in the sample lived near or with their mothers-in-law or mothers, and these older women were a significant source of social and physical support. The depiction of the husband as a caretaker to his pregnant wife in the manual takes the married couple as the central focus of the family rather than viewing the husband and wife as members of an extended family and marks changes that have come to be realized and aspired to in many parts of China. For example, Yan shows that in rural Northeast China young married couples are increasingly forming the center of family life and the son and his wife are replacing the hierarchical tie between father and son. Newlyweds and young people seeking marital partners have formed relationships defined by romantic love, a shared division of labor, and joint decision making, and this has led to a shift in familial power and authority away from parents (Yan 2003). Such changes are entering the realm of pregnancy and childbirth in twenty-first-century China, but in 1994–96, while husbands were providing general physical and emotional types of support, women's female kin and friends formed the core of social support with regard to pregnancy and childbirth.

Chang Guixiang, a twenty-seven-year-old factory worker, proudly announced to me that since she had become pregnant she had not done any housework or cooking. Her mother-in-law, who also works, and her husband had taken over all household responsibilities.

> Sometimes I help out by washing the clothes, but I have not done any housework since I discovered I was pregnant. This is partly because I did not feel well in the first few months; I felt like vomiting and was tired all the time. I am still working, but I come home early because I am so tired all the time. My mother-in-law takes care of all the cooking, and my husband does the shopping. This has helped me a lot.

Xi Jun, a twenty-four-year-old woman who operates a small store with her husband, said that since she became pregnant:

> My husband does a lot more of the work in the store, lifting boxes, moving things, cleaning up. But at home my mother-in-law lives with us, and she takes care of the housework. She is not working anymore, and so she has time. I think I do a lot less work now than before I was pregnant.

Most women at four to six months in their pregnancy were doing some of the daily housework. But, when I asked them who looked after their well-being during this time, twenty-five women first responded that this responsibility fell to their mothers or mothers-in-law. Some mentioned their husbands, but as Sun Limei, a thirty-year-old worker, said:

> They don't know anything about being pregnant. My mother had four children, so she understands and knows a lot about this time. If I have questions, I ask her. She also tells me what I need to eat, and how to take care of myself. She knows what it is like to be pregnant. I don't worry too much because she is living with us now. My husband is OK. He has always been pretty helpful at home; he cooks a lot, but he does not know anything about pregnancy or giving birth! This is women's business!

Sun Limei's comments were ones I heard often from the women in my study. Older female kin reinforced the idea that reproduction is the purview of women, as was made apparent to me when I visited Lu Bin at her home during her ninth month. She and her husband lived with his parents in a two-bedroom apartment allocated by her father-in-law's work unit. Lu Bin met me at the gate of the work unit compound and escorted me to their apartment where her mother-in-law had prepared lunch. The mother-in-law, Yan Renyin, a recently retired high school teacher, served us tea as we sat on an overstuffed sofa in the apartment's small living room. Lu Bin described my research project as one in which I was studying obstetrics and gynecology from a sociological perspective. Her mother-in-law's first questions to me were about my marital and maternal status. Once it became clear that I was neither married nor a mother, Yan Renyin launched into what can only be characterized as a lecture on motherhood combined with a recounting of her reproductive history.

> Being a mother is a natural step in women's lives. When I married, I quickly became pregnant with my oldest daughter in 1964. I was twenty years old at the time and had just graduated from teacher's college in Shenyang. I was assigned to teach at a middle school when I became pregnant, and I taught until my eighth month because there was a shortage of teachers. Life in those times was

much more difficult but in some ways simpler. I received prenatal care at the school's health clinic and was assigned to deliver at a neighborhood hospital. My sister came to stay with me because she had graduated from high school and had not yet been assigned a job. She helped with shopping, cleaning, and cooking. My husband was a machinist in a factory and worked long hours, so when he came home he was not much help. I was not afraid of childbirth because the nurses and doctors at the clinic were very helpful and kind. They went out of their way to make sure we were cared for. If you needed a special test, they would accompany you to the hospital or come to visit you at home in the evenings. My husband was excited about having a child, [and] had hoped it was a son but only because he is the only son in his family.

SG: Did you discuss the pregnancy with your husband at all?

Sometimes, but this is women's business, and I knew that I had the help I needed at the school clinic. I talked a lot with my sister, and my mother [in Harbin] wrote to me with lots of advice about what to eat, what to wear, and not to be afraid of childbirth. Childbirth, pregnancy, these are natural things. But when I went into labor, I had some problems. My blood pressure was very high, and I did not progress into strong enough contractions to move the fetus out of my body. The doctors at the hospital gave me a drug that made the contractions strong but left me weak. In the end, they delivered my daughter with forceps.

As we sat down to eat the lunch prepared by Yan Renyin, she pointed to each dish and told me about its importance in ensuring her daughter-in-law's healthy pregnancy.

See, I have made a fish for us—this is a good source of protein and is easy to digest. Here is a spinach dish, good source of iron; tomatoes and eggs are good protein and vitamins; and OK, sit, sit, you should eat. Nothing is too spicy, it is not good to eat spicy foods when you are pregnant!

Lu Bin laughed softly, and when her mother-in-law went into the kitchen she said, "She is very helpful, but she also likes to eat these dishes! And she worried that you are a foreigner and may not be used to eating spicy foods." Yan Renyin's lunch preparations seemed to be a continuation of how she described her first experience with pregnancy and childbirth, for she was, by cooking an appropriate lunch, caring for Lu Bin. The medical aspects of the process, however, she believed were the purview of medical professionals. At a later meeting with me, Lu Bin said her mother-in-law admonished her to listen to the directions and advice of the doctors and nurses whenever she had a prenatal clinic appointment. Yan Renyin's narrative minimized the participation of the husband in any meaningful way. And later, as we were eating and talking more generally about how China had changed, she suddenly exclaimed that when she gave birth all the physicians in the obstetrics ward were female. The medical staff of the obstetrics department at the Number 35 was also all female, including the physicians. This is not entirely surprising because female physicians have dominated the field of obstetrics and gynecology in China for some time. One day I commented to Dr. Liu as we were waiting for a patient that there were no men in the entire department. She laughed and said, "To have men is not convenient!" Finally, it is interesting to note that when women came to the hospital for prenatal appointments, it was likely that their mother or mother-in-law would accompany them, not their husbands. In fact, I met twenty mothers and mothers-in-law or sisters of the women in my study and only two husbands during my research in the clinic.[11] The divergence between text and practice in this instance tells us that, despite the ideal promoted in the manual, which centered on husbands as caretakers, the logistics of daily life and the patterns of marital residence in Beijing created a situation in which senior women's involvement was still important to these women.

Before turning to the women's hospital checkups and their relations with health professionals, I want to make a few additional observations about the popular pregnancy advice books that women purchased in the hospital and at bookstores. They did not address childbirth, a topic found in popular pregnancy books in the United

States and Europe. None of the other books I purchased at the time in bookstores discusses childbirth in any depth. The two books sold at the hospital (hereafter *Before and After Pregnancy,* and *Complete Book on Pregnancy*) focus primarily on pregnancy, though the former ends with a brief chapter on the postpartum period. The latter explains the signs of premature labor and birth, but the following page discusses the newborn's clothing needs. The final page in the volume lists the things the new mother should have ready to take to the hospital, including infant clothing, pajamas, slippers, sanitary napkins, toiletries, and clothing. Although there is much to say about this phenomenon, the absence of information on childbirth suggests that professionals can best handle this aspect of women's reproductive lives. Indeed, the structure of authority among most women in this study still resided with the older generation and doctors. The books, on the other hand, presented possibilities for a future in which the nuclear family would form the core of women's emotional and practical support during pregnancy. This scenario also supports China's aspirations to modernity through changes in family structure and authority. It reinforces the idea of a modern nuclear family as opposed to the pre-1949 patriarchal and patrilineal family structure that the state has struggled, with only mixed success, to dismantle by means of laws and policies.[12] Such changes could bring about more reliance on expert, professional knowledge rather than that of older female kin since their authority in the family structure will diminish as their daughters and daughters-in-law come to rely increasingly on the marital bond for support. As for husbands, they might be required to participate in pregnancy and childbirth as partners of their wives throughout the process.[13]

Pregnancy and the Prenatal Clinic

For the duration of their pregnancies, care for the women in the study also included the efforts of the doctors and nurses in the hospital. To return for a moment to *Before and After Pregnancy* discussed above, it presents the (male) physician in particular as an important actor in helping a woman through pregnancy and childbirth. The following description of a typical prenatal checkup helps illustrate the ways in which women and medical professionals navigated the encounter and shows us how this moment worked to coproduce ideas and meanings about pregnancy and mothering a healthy child as the mother and physician interacted.

One morning, Lin Xianping, a twenty-four-year-old middle school teacher, arrived at the obstetrics clinic for a checkup. In her sixth month of pregnancy, she was taking time from her school day to come to the clinic. As we sat waiting for her turn, we discussed what she thought about motherhood and pregnancy.

> I like children. I hoped that when I married I would be able to get pregnant and have a child as soon as possible. I worried because my older sister had some problems getting pregnant, and I was afraid I would too. Having children is a natural and normal part of life and makes a couple into a family. Children are a lot of work! I know that I will have to sacrifice some things in my life to raise my child.
>
> SG: What kinds of sacrifices do you think you will need to make?
>
> I will not have time for some of the fun things I like to do. I like to karaoke with my friends sometimes, but with a child I won't have time to do this. I won't spend money on myself the way I can now. If I want to buy a book or a new shirt, I can just buy it without worrying. But once my child is born, I will want to buy things for it. Not just things it needs, like clothing, but there are so many toys and books and things for children now, and I want my child to be able to have these things. But right now I am finally feeling better and have been trying to enjoy myself before the baby arrives.
>
> SG: How have you been feeling? What has changed since we last talked?
>
> I haven't vomited or felt nauseated! I can finally eat food without worrying about feeling sick. There are some things I still don't want to eat, like fish. I feel like my body is getting strong and the

> fetus is growing—look, my stomach is so much larger now! I have borrowed some pants from my husband to wear because I haven't had time to buy new ones that will fit me now. All my clothes are tight, and my body is bigger everywhere. I feel a little clumsy sometimes, and my friends at school tell me I will feel it even more as I get bigger.

The conversation with Xianping before her checkup captures some key changes about what it meant to be pregnant in mid-1990s China. Xianping's observation that children are a natural step for a couple in constituting a family emphasizes the formation of a nuclear family unit—a modern family form to which China aspires using the one-child policy. She anticipated the sacrifice of her newly available leisure time—a result of the state's implementation of the two-day weekend in 1994–95. Xianping also planned to shift the focus of her purchases for her child beyond the necessities—a mark of the unprecedented availability of nonessential goods and a rapidly expanding consumer culture.

When Lin Xianping was called to the examination room, she invited me to accompany her. We entered the room, where a double-sided desk sat between two examination tables. A woman had just stepped off a table and was pulling up her pants and adjusting her clothing as the doctor sat at the desk writing in her chart. Dr. Zhou handed the woman a piece of paper and told her to return in two weeks for her next checkup but to come back if she had any questions or any bleeding or cramping. Nurse Dong ushered Xianping to a scale and recorded her weight on her pregnancy chart. Then Nurse Dong pointed to the exam table and asked her to unbutton her trousers as she pulled a paper roll across the table and tore off the piece used in the previous exam. Xianping stepped up onto the table and lay there waiting for Dr. Zhou. As the doctor approached, she greeted Lin Xianping as Teacher Lin and asked how she was feeling. Xianping replied that she was much better than during her last visit since she had stopped feeling like vomiting every time she ate. As she talked, Dr. Zhou began palpating Xianping's stomach and pulled out a measuring tape, which she pressed to her pubic bone and pulled up over her stomach. As she finished this, Dr. Zhou told her that everything seemed fine and the fetus did not seem to be too large. Xianping laughed and said, "I hope it is not too big because I am afraid of the pain of childbirth." Dr. Zhou patted her leg and told her not to worry, everything was normal. Dr. Zhou looked at her chart and then asked Nurse Dong if Xianping's blood pressure had been taken since it was not recorded. Nurse Dong replied that she had not taken it. Dr. Zhou asked Xianping to sit up, brought a blood pressure cuff to the exam table, and pushed up the sleeve of her sweater to place the cuff around her arm. Xianping noted, "My mother had problems with high blood pressure during pregnancy." Dr. Zhou pumped the cuff and replied, "Your blood pressure was normal at your previous visits. I don't think there will be a problem today. If you are worried, eat fewer salty foods! And come by, as we can quickly check your blood pressure." After finishing with the blood pressure cuff, Dr. Zhou noted that everything was normal. She told Xianping that she could get dressed. Nurse Dong came to Xianping's side as she was stepping down from the table and pulling her pants back up, handed her the pregnancy chart, and noted the date on which she should return for her next checkup. She reminded Xianping that she come in or call if she had any questions. As we left the room together, I asked Xianping if she had ever had questions about her pregnancy and if she did where she sought answers. She replied:

> Sometimes I do have questions about how I should eat or whether I am doing the right things for the fetus. I usually talk to my mother or one of my colleagues at work, but I bought a book here at the hospital, and sometimes I will read it. I know that I can always come here if I have any problems that the doctor might help me with.

Lin Xianping's prenatal visit was typical of many that I observed except that there were usually two physicians seeing patients simultaneously in the room. There was a businesslike quality to the interactions between the staff and women during these sessions. When women expressed nervousness or fear about their pregnancies or birth, the nurse or physician would offer the generic reassurance that everything was fine and not to worry. When women raised specific questions or concerns, however, the staff would respond more specifically as well. In general, there was not always a lot of conversation between the staff member and the woman during the exam. The routine and mundane nature of the prenatal checkup was reinforced by the actions and expected behavior of the pregnant woman during the encounter. There was little small talk during the exam, and women did not completely undress; they simply removed the essential pieces of clothing that allowed the physician and nurse to perform their tasks. Further, simultaneous checkups were occurring on the two exam tables throughout the prenatal clinic hours, so there was no expectation of individualized attention.

The definition of critical moments in the pregnancy when the books suggest that women seek out their physicians did not necessarily coincide with women's opinions about when to see a doctor. One interesting example of this difference is the moment of "quickening" or the time during the pregnancy when the fetus begins to move in the womb. *Before and After Pregnancy* states that between seventeen and twenty weeks the fetus will begin to move (*tai dong*) and that this is a "message" (*xin hao*) to the mother that all is well within the womb. It also emphasizes that the mother should record the date and time when she first feels the fetal movement so that she can tell her doctor (Li and An 1991, 48). Having read this passage in the manual, I expected that women would recall that moment or tell me about it once they had experienced it. Only three could tell me exactly when these began. They did not consider it a particularly important marker of the fetus's development. Perhaps these women's experiences with "quickening" resonate with traditional Chinese medical views that consider fetal movement a not necessarily positive sign. For example, Furth (1987, 13) finds that seventeenth-century medical texts view fetal movement as a dangerous sign of potential miscarriage and that excessive movement required prescriptions for herbs that would act as a calming agent (*an tai*). Women in this study did not view movement of the fetus as a dangerous phenomenon, and certainly it provoked little attention during their pregnancies.

The relative lack of interest on the part of pregnant women with the movement of the fetus was also brought home to me one day as I observed patient-doctor interactions during a prenatal clinic. Dr. Xu asked a woman who was twenty weeks pregnant whether she had felt the fetus move. The woman replied that she had, but she could not remember when it had started. Dr. Xu asked her to try to remember when the movement began three times during the woman's examination, and each time she simply said, "I forget." Dr. Xu later told me that fetal movement can be a sign that the fetus is healthy, but some women did not pay attention to it except to comment that the movements disturbed their sleep or the kicking made them feel nauseous. In this instance, textual information did not translate into women's real life worries and concerns.

Despite the lack of attention paid to fetal movement, women in this study were more conscious of other bodily changes associated with pregnancy. They frequently commented on how large their bellies had grown or how much weight they had gained. These changes were noted because most women feared that the fetus was growing too quickly and would be difficult to deliver. As Ke Hong, a twenty-six-year-old store clerk told me:

> I have gained a lot of weight, and my mother is worried that the fetus is too large. I do not want a large baby because then childbirth will be difficult. So I am trying to eat a little less. I don't want to influence the health of the baby, but I also don't want to have a long childbirth. My mother told me that her births were all very easy because we were all relatively small babies. I hope my baby is not too big!

Zhu Xushuang, a factory worker, often commented on the size of the fetus in our conversations.

> I fear pain. I have always feared pain, even as a child. I know that I will give birth only one time. But it is painful! I watch my belly get bigger and bigger, and I can't stop thinking about how much

> more painful a big baby will be to deliver! There is nothing I can do, but I hope I do not have a big infant.

Here we can see that Ke Hong's and Zhu Xushuang's concern with the growth and development of their babies in anticipation of the pain of childbirth led to different responses. In Ke Hong's case, it was a moment when a pregnant woman's fears conflicted with her duty to nurture the fetus. Her comments indicated that her mother was a critical source of advice and experience about this problem and that, despite her fear of pain, she simply hoped to deliver a small infant; she did not at this point consider taking action to bring about her desire. As the women in this study gave birth and became mothers, we will see that many struggled to balance their needs with those of their infants. For some women, the conflict between their interests and well-being and those of their unborn child began in pregnancy. What is important is that the women responded to these moments in a variety of ways. Some sought to manage their needs as well as those of their infants; others put the infants' needs ahead of their own.[14]

In general, from my observations and interviews, women did not believe that it was necessary to know a great deal about the biological or physiological development of the fetus. As indicated in the description at the beginning of this chapter, during examinations few women asked the doctors about their condition. In one instance, I accompanied a woman named Shi Binyan to an ultrasound appointment in the basement of the hospital, and when I asked her why she was having an ultrasound she did not have a clear idea. She said that the ultrasound had been scheduled to check the fetal heartbeat, but she really did not know any more than that. Her lack of curiosity about why she was having an ultrasound may have been the result of two factors. First, the doctor who scheduled the ultrasound was not very clear about why she needed it. I was in the examination room when Dr. Xu told Shi Binyan that she needed to schedule an ultrasound to check the fetal heart rate, but she said no more and did not offer either reassurances or any indication of what the problem might be. Shi Binyan, as we were walking to the ultrasound room, also said to me, "If there is a problem, the doctor will tell me about it." When we got to the ultrasound room, the nurse adopted a more reassuring stance and said that they were checking to make certain that the heartbeat of the fetus was normal. She told Binyan, "Don't worry, this examination is just to make certain that your fetus is healthy." It was hard for me not to recall an American friend's ultrasound appointments, which the husband often attended, as the couple was well aware of the types of problems the physician was looking for. In the Chinese case, there was little fanfare or concern expressed during the event. The medical staff was not forthcoming about the results, and Shi Binyan assumed that if there was a problem someone would tell her.

While this example was a unique one during my research (few women were sent for such testing), it highlights women's trust that the doctors and nurses would monitor the well-being of the fetus in a medical sense. When I asked women if they had followed the development of the fetus using the pictures of the various developmental stages contained in any popular pregnancy book in their possession, two women told me that they did check a book periodically. Five other women in my sample reported that they had read a book and looked at the pictures early in their pregnancies but subsequently had not used it. The remainder of the sample indicated that they had not yet read any book in depth or at all. As Li Yurong, a twenty-four-year-old office worker in a state-owned company said:

> This [pregnancy] is natural, and I don't think the book can tell you anything that will change the pregnancy. The doctors and Nurse Bai have told me about nutrition, and my mother-in-law cooks nutritious meals for me. So I don't think I can do anything that will influence the fetus except eat well, rest, and not worry.

Although Li Yurong described the course of pregnancy as natural, she was also actively trying to eat well and take care of her body in order to ensure the well-being of the fetus. Her comments also reflect her perception, one shared by almost all the women in my study, that pregnancy is a normal process and not a medical condition. As will become clear later in the chapter, this perspective has changed, and prenatal testing, concerns about high-quality infants, and management of pregnancy as a medical condition have become the norm in the twenty-first century.

Bian Shuli, a twenty-four-year-old cadre who worked at a state-owned publishing house, was one of two women who actively used a pregnancy book to monitor the development and growth of the fetus. She was the most adamant of all the women in the study about the importance of scientific and medical knowledge during pregnancy. This may well be because she was among the most highly educated of the group, with a college degree. She emphatically told me in one of our early conversations that in order "to produce quality infants, it is important to use scientific and medical knowledge during pregnancy and childbirth." Bian Shuli was an avid reader of several pregnancy manuals and asked Nurse Bai and the doctors in the obstetrics clinic more questions than anyone I observed. When asked about what kinds of scientific or medical knowledge were important during pregnancy, she replied:

> Nutrition. This is the most important aspect. Today there is a lot of research on nutrition and eating the proper foods so that you get the vitamins your body needs; this will help the fetus develop and grow into a healthy baby. If a woman, when she is pregnant, does not eat nutritious food, scientific research tells us that the infant may have more health problems; it may be less intelligent. This is also why breastfeeding is important. This is the best nutrition for infants.

Bian Shuli's comments offer a contrast to those who were less concerned about the medical aspects of their pregnancies. The emphasis she placed on good nutrition as a means of ensuring the health of her infant is interesting because this is an action that must be undertaken by the woman herself; it is not something that happens to her. As she expressed later in the same interview:

> I believe that by reading scientific and medical books about nutrition during pregnancy I am helping my child develop into a strong, healthy baby. Only I can influence this aspect of preg-

> nancy. If the fetus has any other problem, that is not something I can influence, if it is a biological problem.

It is also interesting that Bian Shuli assumed that attending to the needs of her body and the fetus during pregnancy required action, so she was proactive about them. She presented a contrast to Huang Fengyi, a twenty-four-year-old woman who owned a small restaurant with her husband and his family. Huang Fengyi's attitude about nutrition during pregnancy was that if she needed to know about it her mother-in-law would tell her. As she put it:

> My mother-in-law tells me what kinds of things I should eat. I don't like everything she suggests or cooks, but she knows what is good. You should eat meat, fish, vegetables, and fresh fruit, and tofu. I know that this is best for the baby, and it is good for my strength, but I do not need to read a book or attend a class to learn this information.

This comment was consistent with many others made by women in this study. The overall message conveyed was that a healthy pregnancy and the healthy development of the fetus depended on the intervention and knowledge of others. Self-knowledge or advice from manuals, such as those sold at the hospital bookstand, was not viewed by most women as important in ensuring the well-being of their infants. Yet a common thread among women's observations about how they thought about and experienced their pregnancies is that the maternal body requires management to support the growth and development of the fetus. This perspective was confirmed for me in discussions I had with all thirty women about the notion of fetal education (*tai jiao*).

Fetal Education

After completing her prenatal visit and breastfeeding class one morning, Bian Shuli and I left the Number 35 Hospital together to shop at a newly opened department store a few doors down the street. The opening of the store was big news in the neighborhood as this was the first such sleek, mirrored, and multistoried department store in the area. With gleaming white floors, glossy photographic images of well-groomed young women suspended over makeup counters full of orderly and colorful displays, and escalators running between its three floors, this department store represented the cutting edge of consumption experiences in Beijing in 1994. On a weekday morning, the first floor was full of people—some strolling and looking over the merchandise and displays and others lingering over particular items as they considered a purchase. We headed for the second floor where clothing and accessories for the family were sold. She had invited me along to check out the shoe selection and the children's department. When we arrived at the children's section of the store, there were racks of clothing for young and teenaged children that obscured a smaller area in a corner that contained infant outfits, blankets, outerwear, rattles, and Johnson baby products. A small display of Qi Qi Tong Fetal Education devices stacked on a shelf caught my eye. The brightly colored yellow boxes featured a cartoon-type drawing of an infant giving the viewer a thumbs up as a globe spins above him. Shuli joined me to investigate the product, and we discovered that it was essentially a small cassette player with "headphones" designed to rest on a woman's belly. Enclosed with the device was a small manual and cassette tape. The idea was to play classical music to the fetus to assist in its development. Shuli was instantly intrigued and decided to buy one for about eight American dollars (I also bought one at a later date). As she stood reading the instruction manual, she occasionally cited the research studies the company had conducted at Beijing hospitals. The scientific evidence of its efficacy appealed to her. The manual noted that with regular usage fetal heartbeats were "calm and steady" and that such states helped with fetal development. It claimed that this modern technology would ensure the birth of a high-quality infant.

Fetal education was not new to Beijing or China in 1994. Despite its modern, mechanized manifestation in the department store, traditional Chinese medical texts of the late imperial period also described the importance of fetal education in ensuring an infant's health. However, the medium of this process in earlier times was the mother's emotional and moral states. As Furth describes it, "Some medical authorities advised a woman to consider her preparation for childbirth ultimately as spiritual self-cultivation." In nourishing the fetus, "[I]f you don't meddle into other people's quarrels, your ch'i will not be injured; if you don't niggle over gain and loss, your spirit will not be burdened. If you are without envy your blood will naturally be sufficient" (1987, 15). According to such traditional texts, the emotional states of the gestating mother were believed to have direct effects on the development of the fetus and could influence the birth and the longevity of the child. The Qi Qi Tong Fetal Education machine represented a contemporary take on fetal education that also required the purchase of a consumer good. After I returned to the department store the following week and purchased it, I brought the device to my next series of interviews and asked the women if they had seen these products in stores and perhaps purchased or used one. Twenty women told me that they knew of or had seen such a product in department stores, but none had purchased or tried one. I found that they all thought it might be a good idea, but it was not something they would purchase because it was too expensive.

I also discovered that a number of popular pregnancy books, including *Before and After Pregnancy*, include discussions of fetal education. The book devotes a two-page section to the concept. Interestingly, it describes fetal education as a tradition hearkening back to an early period of Chinese history and claims that research conducted at that time, and since, demonstrates that fetal education can produce more "civilized" people. It relates this historical authority to the goals of promoting the development and education of children in contemporary China.

> Fetal education can be seen to be important aspects of a good birth and the starting point of good nurturing. In the past, people believed that the fetus before childbirth just quietly slept, waking up only at childbirth. This is a mistake. At three months, the fetus develops a human body, with feelings, and is capable of being

> stimulated by the outer world. . . . At this time you can talk to the fetus. Let it listen to music. Scientific research shows that the spiritual life of the mother and father imperceptibly influences (*qian yi mo hua*) childbirth. (Li and An 1991, 44)

One can see that this statement employs some of the same language and ideas described by Furth in a seventeenth-century text. This contemporary text, however, adds the husband as a factor in the development of the fetus and calls on scientific research to establish that this "ancient" idea has some grounding in the rationality of modern science. It does not specify clearly how the spiritual state of the parents might influence childbirth. Rather, it suggests ways to provide the fetus with a calm, soothing environment. The book also reinforces another facet of potentiality in differentiating understandings of fetal development in the past with those of the present. In the older characterization of fetal development, the fetus was thought to be inert until the moment of childbirth, suggesting that external intervention in its development was not necessary or even possible. The modern, scientific understanding of fetal development, however, makes clear that parents have the ability to influence their future child's well-being.

When asked what they knew or thought about fetal education, a few women in this study were very interested in talking about the way science had discovered how the fetus responds to its environment. But no one clearly linked her spiritual state to that of her fetus and laughed when I asked about her husband's role in its healthy development. The women spoke in general terms about not worrying too much and getting enough rest as the most important ways in which their behavior might affect the fetus.

Despite discussions in the popular pregnancy manuals I surveyed and the availability of the fetal education devices in local department stores, these women were not concerned with this specific spiritual or moral aspect of fetal development. However, the device represents the reinsertion of past cultural values associated with China's own medical tradition into the realm of modernity through technology. In twenty-first-century China, fetal education has undergone some reinvention and modernization. Jianfeng Zhu's recent research (2016) shows that, using neuroscientific knowledge of brain development, the new *tai jiao* (fetal education) represents a more direct attempt by the state to underscore the importance of fetal development during pregnancy. Combining paradigms from biology and traditional Chinese medicine, *tai jiao,* she argues, both reinforces and expands the moral and practical discipline required of pregnant women and serves a larger national project to revitalize traditional Chinese medicine. Zhu finds that, much like the pregnancy books of the 1990s, this contemporary form of *tai jiao* has created a variety of possibilities for women's own experiences and practices during pregnancy. Notwithstanding the apparent differences between women's interests about their pregnancies and those presented in the books, and more recently in Internet forums and television shows, the media do present possibilities and ideals that can be aspired to at the individual and national levels, as becomes clear when issues of population size are considered.

Quality, Not Quantity

The preface to Li and An's Before and After Pregnancy: Remarks on Good Nurturing (1991) places the manual in the context of the larger social and cultural concerns with producing superior babies through the management of Chinese women's pregnancies. One does not need to read beyond the preface to discern this agenda. It begins by stating that China's population is the largest in the world and without attention to the population problem the country's economy, society, and standard of living will all eventually suffer. The book's goals are then set out. It "explains the foundational knowledge of scientific prenatal education, good birth, and good nurturing in helping young mothers give birth to a healthy, intelligent child" (5). The declared goals of the book sound familiar given my discussions in earlier chapters: national interests undergird the focus on individual women's pregnancies, births, and offspring. This particular book, produced by a state-run publishing house, in this case the China Population Press, resembles many on the subject. Publishing houses connected with health, science, and medicine frequently produce such self-help books on a range of topics of interest to the public's health. They are well situated to convey, in both indirect and direct ways, state concerns about a number of aspects of private life. In this book, the science of nurturance during pregnancy is presented as a means of attaining the goal assumed to be shared by the state and mothers: a healthy, intelligent child.

An emphasis on nurture as a responsibility of women during pregnancy is not a recent phenomenon in China. As Bray comments in her work on "reproductive cultures" in late imperial China, "China also had nature-nurture debates, but even in medical representations of fertility and maternity it is apparent that the balance was more heavily tilted toward nurture than ours is at present, and nurture in the social rather than the biological sense at that" (1997, 280–81). While the popular and medical texts of contemporary China emphasize the importance of biology more than those of the late imperial period, there is still importance attached to the nurturance of the fetus as the social responsibility of the mother. The manual's reference to "scientific prenatal education" reminds the reader that the advice presented is backed by the authority of medical science as a symbol of modernity in China. This authority was called to my attention in the first days of my field research when a middle-aged woman who was looking over my shoulder at the Number 35 Hospital's bookstand as I perused this particular book commented, "This is a modern book for modern mothers!" When I asked her what she meant, she laughed and said that when she was pregnant in 1966 there were few books on the subject and women relied on their mothers and mothers-in-law for advice. She noted that now, "Young women don't need the advice of their mothers as they have books, magazines, movies, and television to learn about life." Her comment and the findings of Bray's research help to situate the pregnancy books as presenting new forms of earlier notions about the importance of maternal nurturance of the fetus and as sources of authority that pregnant mothers can resort to outside the influence of their familial networks.

The idea of becoming pregnant for the majority of women in my study was one that they anticipated before they were married. In fact, twenty women told me that once they were married, they immediately applied for permission to become pregnant from the family planning committees at their work unit or neighborhood. As Li Yurong, a twenty-four-year-old office worker for a state work unit told me:

> I wanted to have children as soon as possible after I married, and my husband agreed. We felt that two people in a household are too lonely. A family needs children, or in China, one child. I have never thought much about it; it is a natural part of life. My pregnancy has been fine, no problems.

That the desire for a child is natural was a frequently made point in my early conversations with these women. More important, however, was that the creation of a family satisfied more than just traditions associated with maintaining the family line. Rather, having a child filled in a family and made a couple less lonely.

Yet other women, such as Gu Lijian, who did not want to have a child, mentioned the cost of children in terms of the nation's well-being and their sense that children require attention in order to become properly socialized.

> China already has a large population; we do not need more children. I feel that my work and my husband are enough. Children are expensive and need a lot of attention to rear them, so that they are not "little emperors."[15]

Other women in my study who did desire a child mentioned that China's population problem was related to the traditional desire for a large family. Che Yan, a twenty-seven-year-old store manager, reiterated Gu Lijuan's concerns about population growth but expressed her desire for a child in spite of this.

> China's population is too large. Everyone knows this, and that is why we can only have one child. I think this policy is correct for this stage in China's development. In the future, when China is

> more modern and the population is not growing, people may be able to have two children. I want a child. I did not think much about this before I married, but having a child is a natural part of family life.

The problems of maintaining or developing the "quality" (*su zhi*) of China's population arose in several conversations with women who pointed to rural people as the source of the real problems involved in producing a stronger, healthier, and more intelligent future generation. They frequently referred to rural folks who violated the one-child policy by having two children. Gu Lijuan also raised this issue.

> Rural people, they have no education, and they are having two or some even three children. This is not good for China. How can we become a developed country if the population is so large? The educational and cultural level of these children will also be low. This does not help our country.

The notion that the quality of the Chinese population is directly influenced by excess numbers of people echoes the preface of *Before and After Pregnancy* discussed above. Interestingly, few women at this point in their pregnancies believed that individual women's nurturance of their bodies had the potential to improve the quality of the population. According to most, the problem was overpopulation, caused particularly by the transgressions of the one-child policy among rural Chinese. Implicit in this perspective, however, was the idea that social nurturance is important. Rural people were described as having no "culture" (*meiyou wenhua*), which can mean that they are uneducated or not terribly sophisticated in a broader sense. Such comments suggested that those contributing to China's overpopulation problem were not in the position to raise modern, civilized children. This perception of rural Chinese was not new or exclusive to the problem of overpopulation. It is well known that anyone who is officially, or even perceived to be, a rural resident is considered by Chinese urbanites to be less educated, less sophisticated, and in some sense less modern and worldly.[16]

Beyond the 1990s

My return visits to the Number 35, which continued until 2005, found the hospital in step with the many changes occurring in Beijing's economic and medical milieus. In 2000, the entryway, reception areas, and hallways had been renovated with warm-colored walls and new linoleum flooring. The organization and flow of the prenatal clinic remained the same, but the hard benches where women waited to see a physician or meet with Nurse Bai had been replaced with cushioned chairs. The posters on the walls were no longer handmade but professionally printed, and the chalkboard drawings had disappeared. The messages were the same—eat healthy foods during pregnancy and breastfeeding is best—but the posters looked more like the advertisements found throughout the city, glossy and graphically designed.

Women were still required to attend breastfeeding classes during pregnancy, but Nurse Zhou, a new and much younger nurse, led the class sessions. In 2004, I sat in on a class to observe how Nurse Zhou taught women about breastfeeding. The session was focused on the benefits of breastfeeding—the first session that pregnant women attend. Nurse Zhou introduced many of the same concepts as Nurse Bai, but she emphasized very strongly in repeated statements the importance of producing intelligent children capable of success in twenty-first-century China. There was an emphatic quality to her mini-lecture about how best to nourish an infant. Nurse Zhou noted, "There are no substitutes for breast milk; even the most technologically advanced foreign formula companies have not been able to create a formula equal to breast milk!" She also explained that breastfeeding is a natural and safe way to nourish infants—reminding the women of the many fake products on the market. Nurse Zhou's comments played on very real anxieties circulating in China. Product safety was and continues to be an ever-increasing concern in daily life. Indeed, her comments portended the widespread tainted infant formula scandal of 2008. Single children, with the hopes and aspirations of parents and grandparents riding on their successes in school and work, needed every advantage possible. As one woman in the class commented,

"It [breastfeeding] is such a simple thing to do to help raise an intelligent child! You don't have to buy anything to do it."

Pregnancy embodies anticipation of a future on many levels. From the individual mother's aspirations to the modernization goals of the state, twenty-first-century China reflects an amplification of all the threads found in the Number 35 Hospital and among women in the mid-1990s. Technology, from new forms of prenatal testing to Internet sites with pregnancy advice and discussion forums, is a key driver in this process of intensification in urban China. State policies and rhetoric related to economics and reproduction also continue to shape women's anticipation of how best to nurture and nourish their only children. The stakes remain the same in that women and their families seek to provide the best they can for their children, but the heights to which they must aspire have only increased. The means to help their children have also been commoditized.

Pregnancy, however, has increasingly become a moment of intensified focus in anticipating the birth of a healthy child. In February 2014, the Chinese government announced a halt to all noninvasive genetic testing—especially the prenatal cell free-floating DNA (cffDNA) blood test, which detects fetal chromosome abnormalities and fetal sex. The directive itself made clear the growing popularity of the test since its arrival in China in 2011 (Meng 2014). However, by July 2014, citing high demand for the blood tests that diagnose several genetic conditions, the government reinstated the cffDNA test but under more government scrutiny. A number of concerns underlie these decisions and reflect China's rapidly changing landscape of prenatal care since the introduction of obstetric ultrasound imaging in the 1980s. In 2010, for example, while prenatal ultrasound was widely available, Chinese hospitals had only performed 150,000 amniocentesis tests—a surprisingly small number given the 16 million births that year (Proffitt 2013). I end with these observations because the adoption and incorporation of new reproductive technologies in prenatal health care had not yet reached the Number 35 Hospital in 1994. Concerns about the quality of prenatal care and ensuring the birth of a high-quality child were circulating in formal and informal contexts at this time. Certainly the 1995 Maternal and

Infant Health Law, discussed in chapter 1, represented an expansion of state policy from a focus on limiting births to one of emphasizing the importance of reproductive health care in the production of high-quality children. Infant feeding intentions during pregnancy may well have receded during this shift. Whether it is breastfeeding intentions or prenatal testing, we can see how pregnancy and prenatal care embody a crucial moment in potentials and futures, for the future of the nation and the family rests on the potential child and its mother.[17]

The perspectives of the women in this study remind us that the agents and forms of maternal governance of the mid-1990s, whether derived from prenatal checks, the advice of mothers or mothers-in-law, or popular pregnancy advice books, provided space for different responses from these women. Since then the spaces within which women can maneuver appear to have shrunk. By the end of the twentieth century, policies and trends related to population quality, the one-child policy, and advances in prenatal screening for potential genetic anomalies had raised the stakes for pregnant women.[18]

CHAPTER FOUR

Between Hospital and Home

Childbirth, Infant Feeding, and "Sitting the Month"

Introduction

After the birth of her child, Xi Jun, a twenty-four-year-old clerk in a family store, described her return from a week-long stay at the Number 35 Hospital as part of a process of negotiation between medical personnel and family pressures.

> When I was in the hospital, I still had a lot of blood after the birth. It seemed to be a lot, but the nurse told me it was normal. She and my mother-in-law helped me wash and change the bedding a few times. When I got home, I was so uncomfortable! I just felt exhausted. I could not do anything for the first week I was at home. Breastfeeding was not easy—my nipples were sore and my breasts hurt. Very uncomfortable! My mother-in-law is old-fashioned and made me eat chicken and soup even when I was not hungry. She said if I did not take care of myself now, in the future my body would have problems.

Xi Jun's comments about the early days of her postpartum recovery encapsulate the pressures and dilemmas faced by women in this study once they became mothers. Xi Jun adhered to the goals of the BFHI and breastfed her newborn despite her discomfort. She heeded her mother-in-law's instruction to "sit the month" even while dismissing the advice as outdated. Urban Chinese women expected to observe the long-standing tradition of "sitting the month" (*zuo yuezi*), a one-month period of postpartum rest and seclusion aimed at helping new mothers recover from childbirth. Sitting-the-month practices include staying indoors, resting in bed, and avoiding activities such as showering, drinking cold beverages, brushing one's teeth, and exposing oneself to wind. More than recovery from pregnancy and childbirth is at stake during this moment. Rather, future ailments, as Xi Jun's mother-in-law's message makes clear, may be the lot of women who do not sit the month.

This chapter focuses on the process by which new mothers complied with institutional and informal dictates in order to realize the potential benefit of a healthy child while attempting to attend to their own well-being. Putting up with temporary inconveniences seemed worth the trouble for these women in view of the long-term goal of recovering a healthy body that would enable them to raise a healthy child. From immediately after childbirth to their return home, expressions and expansions of maternal governance appeared medically through the BFHI rules and practices and socially through kinship and the guidance of experienced mothers and mothers-in-laws. New mothers also navigated the feminine ideal of a slim body dictated by their larger social and cultural worlds. While many women internalized these new forms of self-governance, others resisted, finding alternative ideas about how to best restore the postpartum maternal body.

The boundaries between hospital and home, between biomedical and traditional practices, were permeable. Family members brought new mothers, still in hospital, food from home. At the same time, hospitals marketed commercial traditional Chinese medicine products to aid in women's recovery from birth. The BFH, with its emphasis on the importance of producing a healthy infant through breast-feeding, created conditions to further this process: rooming-in with the infant, recovery in private rooms, expert knowledge, and health education. In the postpartum period, then, we can see how biomedical technologies of reproduction in the BFH intersected, and at times conflicted, with those of traditional Chinese medicine and folk traditions. *Recovery,* then, takes on a double meaning. Women literally recuperated from the physical trials of childbirth while recovering possibilities for how best to nurture and nourish their infants from the purview of experts, the technologies of the hospital, and the dictums of female kin.

In this chapter, we first look briefly at the regimens of postpartum recovery in the BFH and how women experienced them. In this institutional space, the routines of the BFHI continued to dominate the parameters of possibilities in feeding the new infant: breast is best. In selections from a detailed timeline of a hospital birth and postpartum recovery, we learn that the goal of successfully feeding the new infant at the breast took center stage. Turning to the home, we look at ideal prescriptions for sitting the month from historical and anthropological sources. These sources offer insight into the parameters of sitting the month and situate the practice in relation to biomedical models of the postpartum body and infant care and feeding in 1990s Beijing. In this context, I then show how individual women's discussions about sitting the month offer insight into how they managed and viewed their postpartum bodies and social relations as they made decisions about breast- or bottle-feeding. We will learn more in chapter 5 about women's decisions about and experiences with infant feeding after birth and on returning to the workplace. The chapter ends by questioning whether and how infant feeding practices of the early postpartum period are being shaped by the development and increasing popularity of private sitting-the month-centers in the twenty-first century. These centers offer women the opportunity, for a substantial fee, to adhere to postpartum recovery traditions under the supervision of a medical staff instead of their mothers or mothers-in-law.

Hospital Births in a Baby-Friendly Hospital

In my observations of six births among the women in this study at the Number 35 Hospital, within an hour of the birth of their infants the women were urged to breastfeed for the first time. This practice fulfilled one of the "ten steps to successful breastfeeding" (see chapter 1) required of hospitals in any part of the globe that want to obtain certification as a BFH. In the hours and days of women's postpartum recovery in the hospital, these ten steps repeatedly touch their lives. In order to facilitate breastfeeding shortly after giving birth, babies are roomed with their mothers, given no water or any kind of infant formula, and are not allowed to suckle on artificial nipples or pacifiers. These practices are designed to establish successful breastfeeding before women return home from their four- to seven-day stay in the hospital, and my study and others in different parts of the world confirm that they generally work well: in my study, all the women breastfed their infants during their stay at the Number 35.[1] The universal adoption of breastfeeding most likely resulted from the support and surveillance of nurses on the ward. The establishment of breastfeeding in any hospital, however, does not guarantee that women will continue after they are discharged, as the next chapter shows. For now I want to emphasize that women, as they recovered in the immediate aftermath of birth in the Beijing BFH delivery room and wards, received instruction and advice about how to breastfeed. The idiom of potentiality continued its presence in interactions between nurses and new mothers as a means of convincing women to continue to breastfeed despite their misgivings or difficulties. At the same time, older, experienced women brought their ideas about how best to care for their new grandchildren to women's bedsides. They, too, communicated assumptions about the potential and promise of each newborn's future.

The following detailed description of these procedures and practices provides a glimpse of the routines I observed in the delivery room at the Number 35 in 1995. Within the small hospital room, once the mother's immediate needs were met, the movements of the midwives seemed choreographed to reach one goal: a suckling infant at the breast of the new mother. The birthing process itself seemed anticlimactic.

> The midwife at the foot of the bed, said to Xuhuang, "I can see its head, just a few more times and you will have your baby!" Once the head appeared and before it actually crowned, the midwife waited for the next contraction and quickly used the surgical scissors to perform an episiotomy. The baby's head emerged and on the following push, the baby slid out very quickly and was handed to another midwife. She immediately put the baby on Zhu Xuhuang's breast and told her it was a girl. The midwife at the foot of the bed waited to deliver the placenta while the third midwife was massaging the new mother's belly very gently to help expel the placenta. The baby, taken from Zhu Xuhuang and examined, was pronounced healthy with the highest Apgar score of ten.[2] As Zhu Xuhuang lay with her eyes closed, the baby was returned to her arms. One midwife stepped outside briefly to tell the waiting family members that they had a girl and everything was fine while the midwife at the foot of the table sutured the episiotomy. Of particular interest here is how soon another midwife positioned the naked baby at Xuhuang's breast, and explained, "Your precious one needs to learn to suckle and needs the nutrients from your breast." Xuhuang held the infant in place and watched as her daughter tried to suckle and within seconds she was nursing. After a few minutes the baby cried and the new mother shifted her position and then seemed too tired to continue nursing.

An obstetrician was never called during these deliveries. When I asked the midwives about this they told me that the physician was only called if the delivery was anticipated to be a complicated one or if any complications arose during its course. The same was true of the pediatrician. However, after the delivery and once the new mother and infant were settled, the pediatrician and obstetrician visited them at least once a day. Otherwise, the midwives ran the delivery room with very little interference from the physicians. The management of labor and delivery by a team of female midwives at the Number 35 offered some continuity with the past in China, where women attended to other women during birth (Furth 1987; Bray 1997; Johnson 2011). This arrangement no longer exists in China. Much as in the United States, doctors now preside over almost all hospital births and therefore represent, in an immediate sense, the medical authority surrounding a woman's birth experience.[3]

Before turning to an analysis of the procedures employed immediately after birth, a few additional details about time in the delivery room will help to contextualize this moment. First, women in labor did not completely undress and don a hospital gown, as is typically the case in US hospitals. Rather, they removed their clothing, usually pajama bottoms, from the waist down and used a sheet to cover themselves. Women did not routinely receive intravenous or epidural pain medications during labor. Pitocin, a hormone that speeds up women's labor, was used on occasion but was not standard procedure. Instead of attaching women to a fetal monitor, as is common in US hospitals, the fetal heartbeat and women's vital signs were checked and recorded at regular intervals by midwives. Finally, no one actively coached or encouraged the laboring woman through her contractions. Nurses and midwives occasionally suggested ways to breathe or grasp the bedrails during contractions, but the women were essentially alone during their time in the delivery room.[4] In sum, childbirth in the Number 35 was a low-technology affair with minimal intervention in terms of medical and social support—until it was time to place the infant at the breast for its first feeding.

At this moment, potential met practice. The information from the prenatal breastfeeding classes taken by these women and the midwives' adherence to the ten steps came together within minutes of the arrival of the infant and its placement at the breast. Feeding the infant was the primary concern while the physical repair and recovery of the mother's body receded to a secondary status. Women at this moment had no choice but to dedicate themselves to nourishing their precious newborns.

The Days after Delivery

New mothers and their infants left the delivery room to recover in either a six- to eight-bed hospital ward with other new mothers or a private room. Private rooms, more expensive than the ward beds, were not covered by insurance and had to be purchased.[5] Indeed, private rooms were a new development in China's hospitals in the 1990s. The Number 35 found that the fees for the rooms helped offset the withdrawal of central government hospital subsidies. In these private but institutional spaces, boundaries between hospital and home blurred as family members, especially mothers and mothers-in-law, stepped in to help care for their daughters and grandchildren. Typically in hospitals, family members supply food and bring items, such as an extra hot water thermos or clean pajamas, that might provide comfort or convenience for the new mother. At the Number 35, infants slept in a small wheeled crib next to the mother's bed. In addition to a bed for the mother and a crib for the infant, private rooms included a bathroom with shower and a reclining chair for family members. According to hospital staff, the private rooms were popular and always occupied. Whether they resided on the ward or in a private room, recovery and potentiality shaped women's experiences in the hospital. During my visits to women shortly after delivery, older female kin were often present. They assisted with much of the practical work of keeping mother and infant comfortable, from changing diapers and bringing food and drink to helping women walk to and from the bathroom and offering advice about how to handle the bodily aftermath of childbirth. When I visited Ke Lin in her private room three days after she had given birth, I found her mother sitting in a reclining chair with her sleeping granddaughter. There was little room for a visitor amid the hospital bed and furniture. Decorated with red—a traditional symbol of good fortune and happiness—with accents in the curtains, a red chair, and a red border around the ceiling, the room felt cheerful and warm. Ke Lin, sitting up in bed dressed in pajamas and a heavy sweater, was eating food prepared by her mother. We chatted about her delivery, how the baby was doing, and her recovery. She recounted:

> We, this baby and I, we sleep and eat and sleep and eat. After eighteen hours of labor, we are exhausted! I have no energy, but I am trying to rest and eat so that my milk will come in. The nurses require us to get out of bed several times a day and walk up and down the hallway—but I am dead tired and have only done so a few times. But my mother has been helping my daughter and me. She brings me lots of nutritious food and takes care of the baby so I can rest.

At this point, Ke Lin's mother interrupts: "You need to rest! When they brought her back from the delivery room, she was shaking so hard from exhaustion. I am happy to hold my granddaughter; I have waited for this day!" Ke Lin smiles and leans back on the pillows:

> I am happy she is healthy. After so many hours in labor of course I am tired, but after one night I already felt so much stronger. My mother is taking good care of us—helping me with the baby and bringing me good food to eat.

After the infant awakens, Ke Lin's mother leans over to adjust the angle of the infant at the breast: "There, she is in a better position so that she won't be at the wrong angle and have difficulty suckling!" Her mother tries to offer me the red chair (I am perched on a small stool), but I suggest that she should rest too since she must be tired. After several attempts to change places with me, Ke Lin's mother sinks back into the chair and says, "I had three children, and I breastfed them all as long as I could. I really had no choice—not like now [when] you can buy infant formula almost anywhere. But I believe that breastfeeding is the best, most natural method. My children all turned out strong, intelligent, and healthy!" The baby starts to cry and seems to be having difficulty latching onto Ke Lin's breast. As her mother returns to Ke Lin's side and helps her position the infant, she reminds her daughter that breastfeeding will take some practice. When I ask Ke Lin how her husband is doing, she replies, "He is so happy! But he has to work, and so he will come and spend the evening and night with us. My mother needs her rest too. At night, the nurses have been very helpful if I have a problem or question. I think it is less busy, so it is easier for them."

Among the women in this study, every one had a family member with her as often as was possible. Those in private rooms were able to have husbands or other family members with them around the clock, but on the wards family members were required to leave by nine in the evening. Husbands tended to come whenever their workdays ended. On my visits, I often found them holding their sons or daughters while their wives slept or rested.

Members of the nursing staff checked on all new mothers and their infants regularly. In addition to checking their vital signs, examining their bodies, and asking questions about their recovery and how often the infant had been put to the breast, the nurses would remind the women that they must get out of bed and walk the hallways every few hours. One issue that several nurses raised was the frequency with which older women would try to get the baby to take a bottle filled with sugar water in addition to the breast. Here we see how informal traditions for soothing and satisfying a hungry or perhaps dehydrated infant clashed with institutional practices. As one nurse noted, "It is hard to help people understand that the baby needs to suckle regularly to bring the milk down and that they can do without water or other liquids from the bottle. I am sure we don't catch all of them, but we try to remind the mothers that there is no need for a bottle." On my rounds with Nurse Bai to visit women after delivery, I noticed that she spent a good deal of time talking about this with families. She often directed her comments to the older women and husbands. She once told me, "Since I am older, I think I can influence the mothers and mothers-in-law by talking to them directly. The new mothers already know that no bottle-feeding is necessary." On her rounds the pediatrician, Dr. Wang, in addition to examining the infant, talked to the family about using the bottle to feed infants. In a very conversational tone, she would remind them:

> "I have taken care of many infants in my work here. We have learned that if we don't give babies a bottle with sugar water they do better in the long run. Their mothers' milk comes in faster,

they learn to suckle properly, and they get the benefits of colostrum from their mothers. We can also see if the infant is having difficulties with breastfeeding and help to correct or improve the situation. Often, once they have been fed with a bottle, infants do not want to breastfeed. So don't worry, we can help you with any problems and make sure that your baby is getting the best nutrition possible."

Dr. Wang and Nurse Bai made certain that, in addition to the new mothers, their mothers, mothers-in-law, and husbands understood the process of establishing breastfeeding. Both women used their experiences and expertise to bolster their authority. Dr. Wang reminded her audience of her long-term experience as a physician. Nurse Bai, in addition to her long experience as a nurse, also knew her age could help her to influence the senior female kin at a woman's bedside.

Recovery and potentiality took on different meanings for both caregivers and new mothers. The nursing and medical staff, in the delivery room and the postpartum wards and private rooms, worked to ensure that infants were born with no complications and were breastfed by their mothers—they were, after all, the guardians of the state's interest in producing healthy and productive future citizens. Older female kin, wishing to secure the well-being of their families' future, also sought to help with the care of mother and child. They provided nourishing and restorative foods and proffered advice about everything from how much exercise women should take in the early days after birth to ways to calm their crying infants and how to care for their postpartum bodies. Mothers themselves were seeking ways to manage their bodies to recover from childbirth and care for their infants. A similar network of negotiation was found by Van Hollen among poor mothers in the days after giving birth in Tamil Nadu, India (2003). She found that tensions between tradition and science intersected with race and class. At this moment in China, however, frictions centered on old and new ways of helping women recover and breastfeed. In sum, the future state that pregnancy embodies had ended with the birth of their children and initiated a new set of potentials and futures for mothers, infants, and ultimately the larger society and state.

Recovery and Potentiality in Sitting the Month

Once women returned home to continue their recoveries, the influence of the hospital appeared to recede and that of experienced mothers and mothers-in-law took over. Women now faced the ritual month-long recovery period during which they were expected to adhere to tried and true practices as a way to regain their prepregnancy bodies and prevent potential health problems as they aged. They also had to balance their needs with those of their newborns. No longer subject to the pressures of institutionalized policies, the women now had the ability to explore alternatives to exclusive breastfeeding. The home provided space, both literally and figuratively, for the advice and experience of female kin, friends, family, and husbands to come to the fore. It was in the negotiations with family in their own homes that women's creative pragmatism also came into focus. To contextualize their experiences, however, let us first look at the customs surrounding sitting the month.

Traditions of Sitting the Month

Thirty days of taboos, prohibitions, and prescriptions grounded in traditional Chinese medicine helped women recover from the trauma and depletion of pregnancy and childbirth. Overseen by their mothers-in-law or mothers, typically new mothers were advised against bathing, washing hair, brushing teeth, eating raw foods or those with chilling effects on the body—and leaving the house. They were admonished to avoid exercise, drafts, and wind (open windows, air-conditioning, or fans). To heal and restore their bodies, they were to eat "heating" foods like sesame oil and black boned chicken, and they must get plenty of rest.[6] Despite the impact of restrictions on their personal hygiene, women in this study adhered to these precepts because they believed their future health was at stake.[7] Many mothers in this study recalled that their older female kin explained their own or other women's ailments as the result of not sitting the month correctly. A friend, Liu Yan, a fifty-four-year-old administrator at a Beijing high school, described the consequences to her health because she could not properly sit the month.

> My first son's birth in 1966 was a difficult one. I had very good care in the hospital, but when I returned home, I only had the help of my husband and an older neighbor woman. My mother could not come to stay with me, and my husband's mother had died many years ago. My mother sent me letters telling me I needed to rest, eat lots of chicken, avoid bathing and brushing my teeth, and avoid going outside or having visitors. My neighbor helped cook nutritious food and even went shopping for us. But my husband was very busy and could not take care of my son or me very much. So I did not really rest. In my old age [she was fifty-four], I have arthritis and back problems. My mother warned me at the time that I would develop health problems if I did not sit the month. She now tells me I would not have had these problems if my husband had helped me more while I was sitting the month. She never liked my husband, so I used to think she was just looking for ways to criticize him. But now that I am older and have these problems, I think that if I had been able to sit the month properly I would be so much healthier!

Women's willingness to believe in the potential to prevent ailments in old age by sitting the month properly is likely reinforced by traditions in Chinese medicine that emphasize the importance of balance between the yang (male, active, hot) and yin (female, passive, cold) in the female body (Holroyd, Lopez, and Chan 2011; Chen 2012). Imbalances of this sort are well understood by most Chinese people as a potential cause of acute and chronic illness.

Traditional Chinese medical understandings of the biology of pregnancy and birth undergird the tradition of sitting the month. In Qing dynasty China, according to Charlotte Furth's research, "Biological processes for women were based on an underlying exchange economy according to which women's vital blood is expended in the reproductive functions of menstruating, gestating, bearing and nursing children" (1987, 28). The blood associated with childbearing was not considered benign. It could pollute and cause illness in the fetus or infant, the mother herself, and her surroundings (29).[8] Yet these potentialities could be prevented by following ritual and medical prescriptions in disposing of the placenta, administering ritual baths, and ingesting special tonics (29). The rest and recuperation of mother and infant for one month away from family and under the care of experienced women formed a crucial requirement to undo the potential for harm and ensure the well-being of the family. The forms of maternal governance of the twentieth and twenty-first centuries, then, have strong antecedents in China's past.

The dangers the maternal body posed to the newborn child's health intersected with the priorities of the family in China's patrilineal and patrilocal kinship system (Furth 1987, 29). Women who married into the family were outsiders and were believed to have the ability to weaken the potential and future of the lineage. The concern was that these wives would hold sway over their husbands to the detriment of his family and lineage. Women thus occupied an equivocal position. Although they were outsiders, their children provided the means through which the lineage could maintain itself. Furth's research shows how medical developments in the Qing dynasty reinforced these patrilineal ideologies (1987, 1999). Qing era physicians sought to safeguard the health of the mother and infant from pregnancy through the postpartum period and in doing so protected the interests of the lineage. Thus, ensuring a good recovery by properly sitting the month served both individual and familial interests.

Patrilineal ideals continue to shape sitting the month in more contemporary times, but these have receded to some extent with the increasing importance placed on conjugal love in a nuclear family.[9] This change has placed new pressures on mothers as they nurture their only children. As part of maintaining their roles as wives and workers, women are also expected to regain their prepregnancy bodies as quickly as possible.[10] These new expectations may be viewed as consequences of a consumer-oriented culture in which women have become both consumers and objects in shaping their lives as mothers (Evans 1997, 1997; Yang 2011; Taylor 2004). In sum, while specific expectations have changed, family futures continue to depend on women's bodily well-being after childbirth.

"I Sat the Month But . . ."

Women's narratives about their actual practices revealed the complex web of considerations in which they made their decisions. Some common themes emerged from their discussions. Most women talked about food, weight loss, relations with their mothers or mothers-in-law, and breastfeeding. Out of thirty women, only one did not sit the month. Zhang Yaoxin, a twenty-four-year-old secretary, told me that she did not follow the tradition of sitting the month. She described her experience during the postpartum period in terms of physical exhaustion.

> My husband cared for me in the hospital after the birth. We had our own room and the baby stayed with us in the room. I stayed in the hospital for seven days. My mother-in-law did not come; she does not live here. My sister came for a few days, but she does not live in Beijing. My mother is dead. I did not sit the month. I think this is a backward tradition. Of course, I did not go out much because I was tired, and there was no need to go out to buy food; my husband did this. I took showers and washed my hair and brushed my teeth. It is not too hygienic (*wei sheng de*) if you don't do these things. I did not sit the month, but I felt a lot of pressure from my [husband's] family to do it. But they don't live in Beijing, and when they telephoned I would not talk to them because the first time I talked to my mother-in-law she put a lot of pressure on me to not read books, watch television. She told me that I would get sick if I took a shower or left the house. I don't believe these superstitions! What could she do? She was not in Beijing.

I asked Yaoxin what her husband thought about the idea of not sitting the month.

> My husband agreed with me. These traditional ways are not scientific (*bu tai ke xue de*), and some are even dangerous! If you do not brush your teeth for a whole month, you can have problems with them later in life. I was very tired after I came home from the hospital and needed to rest. I also made certain that I ate nutritious foods to regain my strength, but I did not drink chicken soup every day as some women do. I did not eat too much because I was still fat from being pregnant. I slept a lot at first and took care of the baby. Breastfeeding was difficult in the beginning, and the baby was hungry all the time. I did not have time to sit the month. I was too busy! My husband took care of me, but he needed to go to work some days, so when I was alone I had to cook, take care of the baby, and try to rest.

Zhang Yaoxin's narrative reveals the importance of a supportive husband and distance from female relatives in her decision to reject "backward" traditions.[11] Yaoxin found that the logic of biomedicine supported her concern that she could avoid future dental problems by brushing her teeth. Indeed, her reasoning in deciding to defy tradition and do things like showering and brushing her teeth also drew on a future-oriented framework of potential consequences.

Although they did sit the month, most women in the study shared Yaoxin's thinking about the consequences of conforming, or not, to this tradition. These women negotiated with mothers and mothers-in-law to find a tolerable blend of practices. Yang Zhiyun, a twenty-five-year-old worker, told me that she had "done the month" in her own way.

> It was hard not to wash my hair. And even though my mother-in-law, who lives with us, told me not to brush my teeth, I did because I felt this was not good. Older people traditionally did not brush their teeth, and now they all have problems! I did bathe with warm water every day. My mother-in-law agreed that since the weather

> was warm and not too windy, it was safe for me to do this. I would have washed anyway. It is not good to wait such a long time to bathe. I did not wash my hair though. It is not good to get your head wet when you are not feeling strong. I ate chicken soup a lot, but no sweets. My mother-in-law made too much food for me every day—I could never finish it all. I did not read books because this can ruin your eyes. I liked sitting the month because I could rest and not worry and take care of the baby. I did not feel too tired after about ten days at home, but my mother-in-law really helped me and let me rest as much as I wanted.

Most women commented on gaining a month of respite from daily household and child care chores as an important part of their recovery. But, much like Zhang Yaoxing, Zhiyun feared that not brushing her teeth would cause future dental problems, and this concern outweighed the potential consequences found in her mother-in-law's traditional knowledge. Du Yan, a twenty-four-year-old office worker, admitted the problems but also the benefits of accepting help from female kin.

> Sitting the month has good and bad aspects. One good thing was that I was very tired when we returned home from the hospital, and having my mother-in-law with us helps a lot. She knows many ways to calm the baby if he is upset or crying. But there are things that are difficult about sitting the month. I am supposed to stay inside for a whole month! I am already wishing for a chance to go outside [she had been home ten days]. My mother-in-law tries to convince me that if I don't follow the rules of sitting the month I will have health problems when I get old. I agree that avoiding wind is important—I don't want to stress my body more. But I should be able to go out to our building's courtyard on a quiet sunny day for a little while. I will probably go outside in the next few weeks after I have recovered some more and feel stronger.

These narratives represent a common sentiment about sitting the month among these new mothers. There were good and bad things about it, and they navigated between traditions and personal preferences to make it work for them.[12] Most women figured out ways to maintain enough of what was acceptable to them within the strictures of the traditional rules. With each rejection of a traditional taboo, however, women reported that their older female kin reminded them of the inevitable health consequences awaiting them in the future. The more difficult struggles revolved around food, eating habits, and weight loss.

Women were simultaneously concerned about eating appropriate, restorative foods and losing weight. Chen Yan, a twenty-six-year-old store manager, expressed these anxieties frequently in our initial conversation after she returned home from the hospital.

> I thought that as soon as I had delivered the baby, I would lose all the weight I gained during pregnancy, but it has not happened! I am trying to eat all the foods I should while sitting the month—my mother is staying with us, and she is a good cook. I want to lose weight, but I know I need to recover. I am breastfeeding my daughter; do you remember how at the breastfeeding classes they told us breastfeeding helps one lose weight? It is not working for me!

During pregnancy, women expected their bodies to grow and were generally optimistic that after childbirth their bodies would quickly return to their prepregnancy shape. Chen Yan's comments noted the failure of breastfeeding to help her achieve her goal to lose weight. This did not stop her from continuing to breastfeed her daughter. Most women anticipated that they would quickly recover their prepregnancy bodies after they gave birth. Han Aihua, an office worker, noted one day during her pregnancy, "It is normal to gain weight right now. I will lose weight after the birth." In the weeks before delivery, many women just could not wait to deliver their babies because they felt tired, clumsy, and awkward. Qu Wen, a pharmacy technician, came to visit me a few days before she was due to deliver. She could not find a comfortable position for sleeping: "I just want to sleep for a night without pain! I wish I could have a cesarean section today just to get my body back to normal!" However, much as Chen Yan laments above, the optimistic view that their bodies would quickly regain their prepregnancy shape diminished for many women after giving birth.

Ke Hong, a twenty-six-year-old worker, although she was happy about breastfeeding in the month after birth and wanted to do the best for her infant by continuing to breastfeed, remained concerned about her weight.

> When will this fat go away! [She puts her hand on her rounded belly.] It has been three weeks since my daughter was born, and I still look pregnant. How do American women lose this fat? I am trying not to eat too much and when I have time I do some exercises that I learned in school, but still I have a big stomach! My clothes from before I was pregnant are still too small. How long will it take to lose this weight?

Ke Hong's impatience about losing weight was about more than body image. While she did worry about her body image, she explained that she would not be able afford new, larger clothes if she did not lose the weight from her pregnancy.[13] Practical matters as much as other pressures weighed on Ke Hong in her quest to lose her pregnancy weight. Six weeks after the birth of her daughter, we met again, and she still felt she was overweight and continued to ask me for advice. While most new mothers voiced concerns about their weight and body shape after birth, few attempted to exercise or diet. They believed that their body was recovering not just from childbirth but from pregnancy as well.[14] One woman, Cui Zhuhong, a twenty-seven-year-old office manager, began exercising as soon as she was instructed to do so by the nursing staff at the hospital. When she returned home she continued:

> "I started to exercise in the hospital—just walking in the hallway. When I got home I felt so weak! I read a magazine article that explained that after childbirth it is not so good to lie in bed all the time. So I started walking in the apartment and doing some arm exercises. But I did not go outside. My mother was already worried

that I was exercising! I will gradually increase [my] exercising as I feel stronger. Otherwise, I feel pretty good!"

The concern about regaining a prepregnancy body shape recalls the image discussed in chapters 2 and 3 of the poster on which an elegant, slim, and negligee-clad mother serenely breastfeeds (see fig. 2). The anticipated future communicated in this image and the breastfeeding class did not mesh with the reality of women's postpartum bodies. The dissonance between the imagined future and the material present contributed to some new mothers' anxieties about their physical beauty and femininity.[15] Yet for others more mundane, practical concerns, such as ensuring that one has clothes that fit and can be worn to work or regaining one's strength after childbirth were more important. The postpartum recovery period brought the materiality of maternal bodies into a new frame for these women as they navigated their recoveries.

In this moment, physically vulnerable, tired new mothers also coped with older women of a generation that regarded eating well not simply as a way to express care and promote healing but also as a recent luxury for Chinese people. Li Yurong's mother interrupted our interview to explain that when she was sitting the month after the birth of each of her three children in the early to late1960s appropriate food for her recovery was a daily uncertainty: "I did not get to eat much chicken after my children were born. It was expensive and not always available to buy. So my mother-in-law made me a lot of dishes with tofu and whatever vegetables were available for sale. We did not have a lot of choices about what food we could buy. Not like these days when you can find anything you want in the markets and stores. They are expensive, but we have more money than when I was a young mother." In the interviews I conducted with women during the first six weeks postpartum, almost every one mentioned the conflict over food and their mother's (or mother-in-law's) authority about appropriate eating.[16] In most cases, women complained that they were being required to eat too much and could not eat everything prepared for them. Sun Limei, a thirty-year-old factory worker, explained during our first meeting, after she returned home, that the picky eating habits that had caused concern during her pregnancy had only continued and indeed worsened while she sat the month.

> My mother-in-law is a very good cook, and so is my husband. But they make dishes that I simply cannot eat—I feel as though I will vomit if I do eat them! . . . My mother-in-law makes me a lot of dishes with chicken—which is fine—but she also uses so many vegetables that I do not like to eat! She tells me they are good for recovering from pregnancy and childbirth, but what good are they if I don't like to eat them? I really like to eat fruit, but I am not allowed to have it for thirty days. My husband has snuck a few oranges and some pears to me at night. If his mother found out, ayahhh! If I have any back problems or arthritis in the future, she will surely blame him. She will blame both of us.

Limei was quite frustrated the day I met with her. She had been sitting the month for about ten days and struggling with the diet provided by her mother-in-law. Limei's husband played the dual role of enforcing the traditions but violating them by sneaking fruit to her. Du Yan also found the amount of chicken she was supposed to eat difficult:

> The baby is fine; he cries a lot, but my mother-in-law tells me that he does so because he is strong and healthy. I am breastfeeding, but it is not easy! My mother-in-law knows a lot about it so she helps me. . . . I am also supposed to eat a lot more food—especially chicken. I like chicken, but my mother-in-law tries to make me eat too much. She says this will help me get my strength back. But I think I will just stay fat, and I want to lose weight now!

Du Yan's narrative ties together concerns about weight loss, difficulties with breastfeeding, and too much chicken. Such difficulties seem distant from older women's postpartum experiences. Yet these new mothers' concerns rested on similar foundations—the importance of future possibilities—those of her future postpregnancy body and the health of her only child.

While the birth of their child formally reconfigured family relations, the demands of sitting the month also changed the family dynamic. Older women, as they oversaw the practical aspects of sitting the month by cooking, cleaning, and caring for their daughters and daughters-in-law and new grandchildren, moved into the center of new mothers' lives. These experienced mothers brought with them their knowledge of sitting the month and the practices handed down by their mothers. Women weighed differently the advantages and disadvantages of sitting the month with the help of their mothers or mothers-in-law. Some women enjoyed the help and comfort of having an experienced older woman to help them and provide them with advice and direction. Others found some of their mothers' ideas to be too traditional or backward and rejected them outright. Ultimately, much as Jianfeng Zhu found in her research among pregnant women and their mothers in Zhengzhou, a dynamic of compromise and negotiation engendered the ways women sat the month (2010).

In some cases, women's relationships with their mothers became a battle over control during the month. Most often these fights and disagreements resulted from the mother believing in the benefits of the traditional practices of sitting the month and the daughter viewing these beliefs as superstitious, harmful, or not very useful. Yan Daifeng, a twenty-nine-year-old factory worker, drew on her status as an urbanite with some education (middle school) in negotiating how best to sit the month with her uneducated, rural mother. She described sitting the month with her mother.

> My mother never had much education. She is from outside Beijing, and she came to stay with my husband and me after I came home from the hospital. She brought three chickens from my parents' house for me to eat. When she arrived, she told me to stay in bed, wrapped the baby in another blanket, and went into the kitchen and started cooking a chicken. My husband offered to help her, but she told him to go watch television and told me that I could not watch it or read books. My friends had also mentioned that it would hurt my eyes to read or watch television. She told me to stay in bed, and she would take care of things. She did all

> the housework, the shopping, and cooked too much food, mostly chicken. Everything was okay, and I learned a lot about taking care of the baby from her during the first week. Then I told her that I wanted to take a shower. I had been brushing my teeth every day even though she told me not to. I just did it anyway. But the shower was different. She told me that too much water on my body would make me sick. She told me that childbirth makes women cold and water is cold and that this would just make me weaker. I think this is just a superstition. But I did not take a shower. I just washed with a basin and a towel.

Daifeng, ultimately capitulated to almost all her mother's instructions. She noted this in a second conversation we had: "I hated sitting the month! I felt like I was in prison and had no control over my life. I did follow my mother's advice because I believed in her ideas but in some cases because I knew from other people that it was okay. In other cases, I thought her ideas were really old-fashioned and backward—not modern or scientific at all. But I did listen to her—she had four children and knows a lot more about this than I ever will." Daifeng's willingness to go along with her mother's instructions came from her trust in her mother's experiences and, in some instances, because those instructions resonated with things she learned from others. She abided by her mother's admonition not to read or watch television because she had heard this from her friends, women like her who lived in urban Beijing. While she followed her mother's rules, Daifeng also differentiated herself from her mother by pointing out her mother's rural background and lack of education. Perhaps because she could see herself as a modern, urban woman, Daifeng could accede to her mother's wishes.

In Xi Jun's case we see how her ability to deal with a difficult mother-in-law came down to using her own money to rear her child as she thought best.

> My mother-in-law and I are not close, but my mother does not live in Beijing, so she could not come until later. My mother-in-law was always telling me what to do with the baby, when I should

> feed it, how I should dress it, but I think many of her ideas were old-fashioned. She also made foods that she knows I don't like because she said they were good for my health. I did not want to eat much, especially at the beginning, but she would leave the food on the table if I didn't try to eat. So I ate a little and then told her I was tired and went back to bed. After two weeks, I wanted to wash my hair. I did not think it was a good idea to wait a whole month. I felt much stronger by this time, but she yelled at me, telling me that I would get sick. The only thing that was making me feel bad was her controlling me!

Xi Jun's story did not end there. She later told me that her mother-in-law wanted to care for her granddaughter when Xi Jun returned to work. Yet Xi Jun had already decided to find a nursemaid (*bao mu*) rather than let her mother-in-law take her daughter every day. She said, "The *bao mu* may have some backward ideas because she is from the countryside, but she will listen to me because I pay her salary and give her a place to live. My mother-in-law will never listen to me." The issue of child care is discussed in the next chapter. However, here it is important to note Xi Jun's feeling that she did not have control of her life in the early days after childbirth. Her description of that time also reveals that while she believed her mother-in-law's help was necessary at that point, it still made her feel helpless. She responded by planning for the time when she would need child care, circumventing her relationship with her mother-in-law, and hiring a nurse. Women's relations with their mothers and mothers-in-law while sitting the month highlighted the contingent nature of kinship relations and gender roles. This conclusion echoes with Gammeltoft's finding that in Vietnam decisions about whether or not to continue a pregnancy rest with both Vietnamese women and their families. In making such a decision together, women reaffirm their membership in their husband's kin group (Gammeltoft 2014, 206). Yet, while sitting the month reinforces the cultural ideals of China's patrilineal kinship system, the women in this study drew on their positions as educated, employed, urban, and modern individuals to navigate these social relations.

When it came to supporting breastfeeding and caring for their infants, most women appreciated the experience and knowledge of their mothers and mothers-in-law. Shen Jun, a twenty-four-year-old woman, described the way her mother cared for her newborn twenty-four hours a day. She had only been home for about five days, but her mother quickly established the routines necessary to care for mother and infant.

> My mother has taken care of our "precious one" (*baobao*) since we came home from the hospital. I breastfeed her, but she takes care of her most of the time, especially when I am sleeping. My mother, the baby, and I are all sleeping together in one bed. If the baby wakes up during the night, my mother checks to make certain it has not urinated. If she discovers that the baby needs to be changed, she gets up and does it. If the baby is hungry, she will place her next to me so that I can breastfeed without getting up.

Shen Jun's mother interjected a comment at this point in our interview, pointing out that she had taken on these responsibilities because she wanted to make certain that Shen Jun focused on her own recovery: "Shen Jun's labor was a long one. Not like me; I delivered my three children very quickly. Childbirth is exhausting, especially when it takes such a long time. I want her to rest as much as possible so that she can regain her strength, make sure she has plenty of breast milk, and avoid future health problems." Mother and daughter believed that breastfeeding is important. Shen Jun appreciated the work her mother had taken on and, of all the women in this study, seemed least concerned about adhering to the traditional taboos of sitting the month—she saw them as important to her recovery.

The lack of bodily control experienced by some women as they tried to breastfeed during the month clarified for Bian Shuli the necessity of shifting to infant formula. A manager in a state-owned publishing company, Shuli's experiences with breastfeeding and the bodily changes that occur after birth overwhelmed her.

> In the hospital, I had no milk until the third day after I gave birth to my son. I tried to feed him before that, but there was no milk, and he just cried and would not suck. When my milk did come, it came all the time! Because the baby was in the room with me, every time he cried, milk would start pouring out of me. The nurse told me that this was good because I would have plenty of milk and could breastfeed without any problems. But I was also uncomfortable after the birth; I was tired. The milk just made a mess; blood, milk, I felt like things were just coming out of me all the time. When I got home, I knew that I should breastfeed, and I did for about two weeks. But it was too messy, and I knew that I was going to go back to work in a few weeks [six weeks after the birth], and I just could not have milk coming out of me at work. I also knew that I would be leaving the baby with my mother-in-law during the day and would not be able to breastfeed during the day, so I started mixing breastfeeding with infant formula. I use a foreign formula and started adding a bottle at night. My mother-in-law agreed that it would be better to get my son used to the bottle right away. My milk has stopped, and when I go back to work in a few weeks I won't have to change my shirt three times a day!

Shuli was concerned with leaving her son and not being available to breastfeed when she returned to work. Her description also indicates that she felt messy and had no control over the breast milk and body fluids that continued after the birth. She managed the breast milk leakage by switching her son to infant formula soon after she returned home.[17] In this case, Bian Shuli felt that she needed to regain her prepregnancy body in anticipation of returning to work, where she believed she would face an uncomfortable and inconvenient struggle with breastfeeding during the workday. The next chapter takes up how women anticipated their transition to work and sought practical solutions so as to provide the best for their children.

Conflict and disagreement between the two generations, however, almost always led to a compromise over how best to sit the month with little long-term fallout between the two generations of women.

Jianfeng Zhu's study (2010) reinforces this finding. Her research in Zhengzhou documented middle-class mother-daughter negotiations about the relative merits of consuming nutritional home-cooked foods versus scientifically produced vitamins and supplements during pregnancy. She found that these negotiations were often heated but that the conflicts resulted in compromise and also served to reinforce the importance of the women's relationship rather than diminishing it. Zhu suggests that we might consider mothering in China as a hybrid and dynamic process that engages state interests alongside those of the mother-to-be and her mother or mother-in-law. Her work also makes clear that caring may reveal itself in conflict rather than patience and nurturance (419). The negotiations between new mothers and their mothers or mothers-in-law about how to eat during pregnancy or how to sit the month remind us that patrilineal family structures and expectations were still present in the 1990s (as they continue to be). Just as we learned that some women's compromises with their mothers-in-laws about having a child at all reflected long-standing practices, it is likely that negotiations about how to sit the month were also not necessarily new. Finally, these negotiations remind us that concepts of individual choice and control in understanding reproductive decisions may not best represent what happens as women sit the month and feed their newborns. Perhaps we should invoke the framework of "obligatory choices," the term used by Elly Teman and her colleagues to better understand that when dealing with questions about the use of reproductive technologies, ultra-Orthodox Jewish women exercised their agency without drawing on considerations of individual choice. In their study, they found that as women navigated prenatal care and testing they faced a paradoxical situation in which they believed that the outcomes of their pregnancies were predetermined by God and yet they were obligated to make an effort to prevent problems and facilitate the birth of a healthy infant (Teman, Ivry, and Goren 2016, 284). Though certainly not directly parallel, Chinese women made obligatory choices in the face of traditional wisdom about how best to recover their bodies from the stresses and strains of pregnancy and childbirth and ensure their long-term health.

When it came to figuring out the best way to feed their infants, less negotiating between the two generations of women occurred. In part this may be attributed to the success of the BFHI. New mothers had received an education on infant feeding grounded in the authority of science during their classes at the Number 35. This knowledge, as well as the practical concerns about returning to work, seemed to give them the upper hand in making infant feeding decisions.

Sitting the Month and Infant Feeding in the Twenty-First Century

In August 2015, a new mother in Shanghai died while sitting the month. Fearing the effects of cool air and wind, in the heat of summer she kept herself wrapped in a heavy quilt in a room with closed windows and no air-conditioning. This mother's death followed another in which a woman died of a pulmonary artery thrombosis after not moving about her apartment while sitting the month (*China Daily* 2015). These events sparked widespread debate in China's blogosphere about the relevance of sitting the month in the twenty-first century (Fan 2015). While many question the value of sitting the month, others defend the practice, citing the potential short- and long-term health consequences. A 2005 survey found that women throughout urban and rural China continued to sit the month and many adhered to some of the long-standing traditions: more than 70 percent of women did not wash their hair and almost 40 percent did not open windows in order to avoid wind (Li, Zhang, and Dong 2005). The persistence of these customs, as evidenced in the popularity of sitting the month centers and debates in the blogosphere, cannot simply be explained by the power and authority of the older generation over new mothers.[18] Rather, the future health and well-being of mothers and their single children rest on a successful postpartum recovery.

Should women sit the month using modern, scientific methods with the assistance of experts or is it something women should do at home under the care of their mothers-in-law or, better still, their mothers? These debates are linked to recent technological and institutional developments in the context of China's increasingly medicalized and consumer-oriented society. Beginning in the early twenty-first century, sitting-the-month centers or hotels have opened in China's major cities. These centers offer the opportunity to sit the month under the guidance of physicians and nurses, allowing new mothers to recover from childbirth away from the purview of their mothers-in-law and/or mothers.

Such services and amenities come with a high price tag. A one-month stay at the most luxurious center in Shanghai, for example, costs US$27,000 (Levin 2015). Rates include a room on a par with one in a five-star hotel, a special postpartum diet based on traditional Chinese medicine and western science, twenty-four-hour nursing care with four caretakers per new mother, physicians on call to care for mother and infant, exercise classes, a beauty salon and spa, and weekly checkups with a physician. In one center, women are also bathed weekly by two trained nurses using a traditional Chinese medicine decoction. In 2014 families in Zhengzhou, the capital of Henan Province in central China, could expect to pay an average of ¥10,000 (US$1,650). Despite the costs, centers are fully booked and have waiting lists (Zhao 2014).[19] As urban residents' average annual per capita disposable income in 2013 was ¥26,995 (US$1,644), a month-long stay at a maternity hotel represents a substantial financial investment (Zhao 2014). Whether women sit the month in such luxury or at a more modest center, the primary goal of the staff is to ensure that women follow the rules for a full recovery from the burden of pregnancy and childbirth.[20]

What happens to breastfeeding in such an institution? In visits to two centers in 2004 and 2007 in Shanghai, as well as in blogs and new reports, I found that breastfeeding seems to be promoted and supported by medical staff. Indeed, women are fed special soups and tonics that help with breast milk production. However, most infants are not roomed-in with their mothers twenty-four hours a day. The centers I visited offered the option of having the baby in the mother's room during the day, where she could breastfeed on demand, or she could have the child brought to her for breastfeeding on a regular schedule. Infants, however, spent the night in a nursery where they were bottle-fed by the nursing staff. Despite what many breastfeeding experts would consider less than ideal circumstances, the message women receive at these centers is that breastfeeding is the most scientific and natural way to nourish their precious only child. With such hands-on care, women who stay at these centers likely receive a good deal of breastfeeding instruction and support. How such support translates into sustained breastfeeding has yet to be determined.

Whether it is 2015 or 1996, women's postpartum recovery and the nourishment of their children rest on potentialities. These potentials, as we have seen in the ways in which women navigated the tradition of sitting the month, are shaped by tradition, science, consumer culture, and the interests of the Chinese state. These new mothers' responses and practices make visible some of the agents of maternal governance—both new and old—as well as their creative responses. For women, their immediate and long-term bodily well-being is at stake. In the most direct sense, women seek to ensure their health by following the traditions of sitting the month. As they balance the demands of postpartum recovery with their decisions about how best to feed their infants, they are also managing their families' future well-being.

CHAPTER FIVE

Maternal Maneuvers

Between Home and Work

Introduction

Women's recovery at home while sitting the month and their eventual return to work marked a time of transition when the earlier potential future of their pregnancies met their present realities as new mothers. On another level, the weeks and months after women returned home from the hospital tested the potential of the BFHI to increase the number of women who would exclusively breastfeed. Would the rules and routines—from prenatal breastfeeding classes to adherence to the ten steps after childbirth along with the support and advice of trained health professionals—be enough to encourage all thirty women to breastfeed exclusively for four to six months? This chapter looks at the infant feeding decisions women made during the four- to six-month postpartum period as these new mothers navigated their worlds and resumed their work and family life in a rapidly changing economic and social milieu.

The move from home and hospital certainly allowed women more freedom to maneuver between outside pressures and their own desires. After sitting the month, these new mothers resumed sexual relations with their husbands, returned to work, and cared for a rapidly growing infant. Some heeded the hospital's message that breastfeeding represented the best hope for rearing a healthy, intelligent child while others found that infant formula or a mix of breast and bottle-feeding best served their infants. All were aware that the consumer culture of urban Beijing idealized the sexualized female body. They also faced a work environment in which motherhood was increasingly considered a liability. In the accounts that follow, we see a crosscutting of values, ideals, and power relations complicating women's lives as they worked out their myriad responsibilities to the nation, the family, their husbands, and their single children alongside their personal desires.

Before turning to women's narratives about the ways they managed competing demands at home and work, we first look at the role of women's work in China's recent history alongside research on infant feeding practices around the world. Paid employment in women's lives has long formed the basis for policies about how best to bring about gender equality. Grounded in Marxist theory, the state enthusiastically embraced the logic of liberating women by bringing them into the labor force from the earliest days of the founding of the People's Republic of China in 1949.[1] Many readers will be familiar with Mao Zedong's famous statement about gender equality: "Women hold up half the sky." China's success in women's employment is noteworthy; by the late 1970s, more than 90 percent of urban women were working (Bauer et al. 1992). By the twenty-first century, however, there were dramatic declines in urban women's employment. This decline was accelerating at the time the new mothers in this study were returning to work in the mid-1990s. At the same time, research around the world was demonstrating that women's work outside the home deters exclusive breastfeeding (Nerlove 1974; Rudzik 2012). Long working hours, commuting, and lack of on-site child care are often cited as reasons for the incompatibility of breastfeeding with women's work. Work, then, stands at the intersection of these two policy and research agendas.

As we will learn from their narratives later in the chapter, almost all the new mothers held work central to their lives, which required balancing the needs of family with the demands of their jobs. In this balance, women must weigh the potentials for both mother and child. Could mothers endure the process of breastfeeding while working? Would their needs and those of their infants be best met by breastfeeding only to the end of their maternity leaves? These women's consideration of such questions, along with others, reflects calculations encompassing both the present and the future. Within these deliberations, we will see the ways in which the reach of the BFHI extended—or not—to these women's lives as they returned to their work.

Women and Work in 1990s China

Two terms related to work in mid-1990s China circulated in the worlds of the new mothers in this study and likely shaped their infant feeding decisions. The first, *xiahai,* literally means "to enter the ocean," but colloquially it refers to taking the plunge into finding work in the new and risky private sector. It meant that one was giving up the "iron rice bowl," a job in a state-owned enterprise (*danwei*), which provided workers with such benefits as subsidized housing, child care, health care, education, and pensions. The other phrase, *xiagang,* translates as "laid off from work." The number of laid-off workers in urban China accelerated as state-owned businesses began losing subsidies and support from the government as part of its efforts to restructure the economy from a socialist to a more privatized capitalist one—market socialism. As a Chinese friend of mine, using a reproductive metaphor, put it, "The umbilical cord has been cut, and now each work unit must breathe on its own!"

Women bore the brunt of this restructuring in a number of ways. By 1993, a survey of seven provinces in China found that 60 percent of those laid off were women (Meng 1995). Women's precarious employment situation began in the 1980s, as state-owned enterprises looking to lay off workers began offering women extended maternity leaves at reduced or no pay (Jacka 1990, 2). A number of women in this study were offered the opportunity to extend their state-mandated, paid, ninety-day maternity leave for a year, or in some cases two years, at reduced pay. No one planned to accept this deal. Every woman offered this plan was aware that if she took an extended maternity leave she was not likely to return to a position in her work unit. These women also worried about making ends meet. As Ke Hong, a store worker, commented, "We cannot afford a long maternity leave at only half of my salary. How would we have enough money to live, and with the baby we will need more money not less!" As we will see in the narratives below, women's anxieties surrounding a changing employment landscape surfaced most acutely during the early days and weeks after the birth of their children.

Over two-thirds of my sample worked in state-owned or collective enterprises, but seven women worked in small family businesses or *getihu*. While many people at this time were considering leaving their jobs for the private sector, these seven women were laid off from state companies and had started small businesses, in some cases joining forces with other family members and in others operating on their own.[2] These businesses were service oriented and included three women who worked as tailors/seamstresses, one woman whose family ran a copying and printing store, a woman who had a small convenience store on the street in front of her apartment building, and a pearl seller at a local pearl market. These women had some security in that they received subsidies for health insurance and other services from their former work units. But their livelihoods as small businesswomen depended on their labor. Five of the six women had husbands who worked in state-owned businesses or for the government, so they had some economic security. But they were all too aware that the iron rice bowl could easily disappear for their husbands. I intentionally created a sample that would include these women because I was interested in learning whether they might make decisions with regard to infant feeding different from those of women who worked in formal jobs. As we will see, the nature of the business and the support of kin played important roles in the way this group of women fed their children. Whether formally or self-employed, women in the mid-1990s faced a great deal of economic uncertainty when they became mothers, and this uncertainty was one factor in the decision to either breast or bottle-feed.

Although socialist supports were disappearing in urban enterprises, socialist notions of the ideal woman as a contributor to the labor force continued. Female participation in the labor force in China has long been one of the highest in the world. In 1990, for example, almost 90 percent of urban women between the ages of twenty-five and forty-four were employed (Wu and Zhou 2015; Bauer et al. 1992).[3] These rates reflect in part the legacy of policies and campaigns implemented by the CCP after 1949. Indeed, during the Maoist years (1949–76) a number of protective policies for women were instituted as a means of ensuring urban women's participation in the work force. The CCP's political stance and authority rested in part on Marx's and Engels's assessment that only when women are incorporated into the work force and have access to their own means of support will equality between men and women be achieved (Honig and Hershatter 1988). The Chinese state, particularly in the 1950s and 1960s, emphasized that women's domestic responsibilities prevented them from achieving liberation and equality. Government campaigns promoted the socialist woman as a worker by identifying and publicizing model women workers. Most well-known to westerners are the "iron girls" working in typically male professions such as welding, mining, or construction in an effort to effect normative changes in Chinese women's roles (Robinson 1985; Evans 1997). During the collective period beginning in the late 1950s, efforts were made in some places to remove women's domestic responsibilities, such as cooking and child care, from the family by establishing communal canteens and child care centers so women could focus on productive work for China's modernization. Women's labor thus came to embody a moral value as exemplified by Jacka's findings that in some contexts women who were overly concerned with their household duties were considered selfish (1997, 35).

Although the canteens and child care services were short-lived, paid maternity leaves, nurseries in the workplace, and menstruation leaves were benefits available to many women in urban work units. But, as these began disappearing after 1978 when factories and enterprises sought to make a profit under the market reforms, Margery Wolf found that factory managers were "afraid of having to add special facilities, such as nurseries, and they assume that the factory would be less efficient because of women's 'special problems'" (1985, 60). The consequences of these changes in terms of women's work meant that women were increasingly viewed as troublesome employees because of their reproductive responsibilities (Wang 2003, 166). The pressure to increase efficiency and cut costs in state-owned enterprises accelerated in the early 1990s. Urban women seem to have borne the brunt of the massive restructuring of China's economy. Census data from 1990 and 1996 show that women's employment had declined by almost 10 percent. By 2003, when the restructuring ended, women's labor force participation had reached a low of 63 percent (Wu and Zhou 2015, 320). Despite these trends, or because of them, women in this study valued their work outside the home.

Lisa Rofel's research among three generations of women factory workers in the 1980s, however, shows us how different generations identified with their work in ways that reflect broader historical moments in modern China. She found that the oldest generation's ideas about their work lives resonated with the CCP's efforts to liberate women. They were provided with the political and social means to work outside the home and perform the kind of work that had typically been assigned to men. The youngest cohort, however, found less meaning in their work lives and sought to fashion identities grounded in domesticity and motherhood (1999, 192).

While the women in my sample were navigating a world that increasingly emphasized ideals of femininity and domesticity, they worked for economic reasons and their independence. Eighteen women in my sample declared outright that the work site was the only place where they could escape from the demands of their households. Even if they were not particularly happy with their jobs, most women wanted to continue to work. The connection between autonomy and work resonates with what Wolf found of urban Chinese women in the 1980s: "Without a [work] unit of their own, they remain children of their parents, receiving from them their rations, their pocket money, their identity" (1985, 60). It should come as no surprise that women, as they became mothers in 1990s Beijing, were faced with a complex set of demands, for they had to be at once good wives, nurturing mothers, and productive workers in an uncertain economy. The following section examines the ways in which women expressed their feelings and experiences with physical bodies that were now supposed to be nourishing a baby and returning to a pre-pregnancy shape. As these women moved on with their lives, they were constantly reconfiguring their bodies, bodily functions, and social relations.

Infant Feeding beyond the Mother-Child Dyad

All twenty-nine women, after their first and third breastfeeding classes, planned to breastfeed. A few women admitted they would do so only for a few weeks.[4] These women expressed worries about weight gain, sagging breasts, and messiness. Over half the group feared that breastfeeding would tie them too closely to the baby and prevent other family members from helping to care for the child. These women, as they awaited the birth of their children, anticipated that they would be balancing the negative and positive aspects of breastfeeding in their own lives. At the same time, they wished to do everything they could to raise a healthy and intelligent child.

Before moving on to women's discussions about their decisions, figure 3 indicates the number of women breastfeeding, bottle-feeding, or mixing the two and provides a summary of these practices at two points in time. Specifically, in the first six weeks after the birth of their children, twenty mothers had switched to a feeding regimen that included infant formula. Of these, twelve were using infant formula exclusively. We can see that by four months, seven women were exclusively breastfeeding, thirteen were exclusively bottle-feeding, and ten were mixing the two. However, discussions with women about their reasons for choosing these infant feeding methods reveal complexities about these decisions that are hidden if one relies solely on a chart. For example, at the six-week interval, four women were primarily breastfeeding with an occasional bottle of infant formula used when they were away from their children. They had begun this practice in the first month after birth. Other women found breastfeeding problematic at some point and decided either to switch to infant formula or to mix breastfeeding with bottle-feeding. The chart, and the data that constitute it, present a static view of an evolving decision process. In practice, however, we can see how the potentialities of infant feeding practices met the fluctuating realities of these women's lives. Their narratives reveal that the course of action taken resulted from those forms of agency available to them in the face of constraints imposed by the changing importance of work, kin relations, and marriage. This point bears close attention because public health research, policy making, and program designs seeking to promote exclusive breastfeeding use such cross-sectional findings both to document barriers to breastfeeding among wage-earning women and to measure the success or failure of initiatives meant to promote increases in rates of breastfeeding.[5]

At another level, epidemiological measurements of rates of breastfeeding contain a mathematical logic that brings order to our understanding of women's infant feeding decisions. The process of categorization of individual women in terms of whether they conform or not to established medical views that deem exclusive breastfeeding a healthy behavior situates mothers in a familiar framework of rationality and, by extension, morality. It assumes that individuals will seek to maximize their desire for a healthy infant by making the rational choice to breastfeed. Those who choose alternatives to breastfeeding, by this logic, are not acting in their infants' best interests and thus are making irrational and ultimately immoral choices. What kind of mother would put her child's health at risk? As becomes clear in the women's own words, infant feeding decisions are always rational, but it is a rationality that depends on context and thus is not easily generalizable. Among those women who switched to a mixture of breast milk and infant formula during the first six weeks after the birth of their children, Lu Bin, a twenty-seven-year-old publications manager at a state-run publishing house, tells how she managed to find a solution that rejected the authority of her mother-in-law in favor of a foreign product.

> I know that breastfeeding is best for the infant, but I had trouble with it. At first I did not have any milk, so when I put my baby to

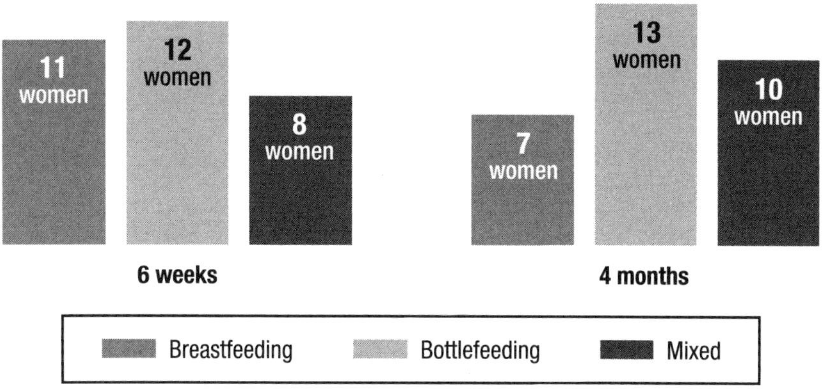

Figure 3. Mothers' infant feeding methods at six weeks and four months

my breast, he sucked and sucked and nothing came out so he would start to cry. He would not stop crying because he was hungry. For the first four days in the hospital nothing but colostrum came out of my breasts. The baby was so unhappy because he just did not have anything to eat. Finally, on the night of the fourth day, my milk started to come in and at first I had a lot of milk.

When I returned home from the hospital [after seven days] my milk did not seem to satisfy the baby. I was feeding him every hour sometimes, and after he had breastfed he would just cry. I think that I did not have enough milk to make him full. My mother-in-law thought that I needed to eat more and made me all kinds of foods, including lots of chicken and some herbs to help strengthen my blood and thus increase or improve my milk. I am still not sure whether I did not have enough milk or it was not good enough.

Finally, four days after we came home from the hospital, my mother-in-law gave him some boiled cow's milk. He drank the milk and went right to sleep. This was the first time he had done this! I think my milk was not enough for him; it did not fill him up. So, I decided that I would keep trying to breastfeed but I would also give him some infant formula. I did not want to use cow's milk because it is not safe for infants. I bought a foreign brand of for-

> mula and now [at six weeks] I feed him twice a day with formula and breastfeed at other times. This has really been a very good method for me. He sleeps and does not cry so much and I can rest.

Lu Bin's distress about her baby's reaction to breastfeeding made me wonder about expectations for infant behavior and breastfeeding. Her narrative took me back to the breastfeeding video discussed in chapter 2. Reviewing it again, it is striking that when newborn infants appear in a scene with their mothers they are either breastfeeding or sleeping. In fact the video shows one new mother trying to keep her infant awake while it breastfeeds. It is certainly too simplistic to directly link Lu Bin's viewing of the video and her expectations that babies should eat and sleep with little crying in between these events. However, the video, Lu Bin's expectations, and her mother-in-law's observations converge around the idea that a crying infant is not satisfied with its mother's milk.

Lu Bin's response to her infant's behavior contains a logic that might be dismissed by contemporary health experts as an incorrect one. Scientific evidence suggests that, except in extreme circumstances, all women can produce adequate breast milk.[6] Yet her attempts to remedy the deficiency in her breast milk by improving her diet and eating foods that would strengthen her blood mirrors Qing dynasty medical conceptions about breast milk and may be viewed as a translation of the historical expertise of traditional Chinese medicine into the modern context. Charlotte Furth's research indicates that breast milk was an important aspect of women's relationship with their infants' well-being.

> Infancy continued the symbiosis between mother and child through the bond of breastfeeding. Medical authorities liked to see weaning delayed until a child was past two (three sui).[7] In the traditional medical view, breast milk is literally transformed yin blood, which manifests itself first as menstrual flow, then as the placental blood nurturing the fetus, and which after birth rises through the mother's body in the form of milk. Once again the mother's responsibility for the health of her infant was medically

> emphasized, because lactation, like pregnancy, has a direct physical impact on the child. Proper diet and conduct and the regulation of sexuality and emotions were the key to keeping the milk wholesome and the child well. (1987, 22)

More contemporary, popular manuals do not describe the symbiotic relationship between mother and child specifically in terms of the traditional Chinese medical concepts of yin and yang, but they do make similar connections between the mother's regimen and the quality of her milk. For example, a 1992 manual titled *Ren Shen Yu Fen Mian Da Quan (The Complete Book of Pregnancy and Birth)* emphasizes the importance of the mother's nutritional and emotional states as a necessary correlate to successful breastfeeding: "The mother who has just given birth still needs to think, as before the birth, to take care in her lifestyle, to follow a regimen, get enough sleep, be in happy spirits, [as] all these things can influence milk secretion, causing insufficient milk" (Du 1992, 55). The manual also spends some twenty pages outlining the different nutritional requirements of the nursing mother and child during the first six months. When mothers like Lu Bin react to their infant's behavior they are also responding to a broader cultural milieu that emphasizes an embodied maternal responsibility for these behaviors.

Zhu Xuhuang, a twenty-four-year-old factory worker, described similar difficulties and gave her reasons for switching to infant formula.

> I had a Cesarean section because the doctors decided that the baby was too large for me to give birth. After the operation, I was very weak and tired. My milk was influenced by the surgery. I tried to breastfeed in the hospital, and the nurses helped me during my stay, but it was uncomfortable to nurse with the wound on my stomach. I breastfed in the hospital, but when I returned home, my milk was not sufficient. The baby cried so much, and every time I tried to breastfeed, she would cry and I cried too. Finally, I realized that I was exhausted and my body was not able to produce enough milk. My mother was staying with us, and she suggested that I try using infant formula. Once I did, the baby was sleeping

more and not crying so much, and I felt better too. I could rest my body and build my strength.

Zhu Xuhuang's decision to switch to infant formula reiterates concern about the appropriate responses from an infant, which reassure a woman that her body is adequately nourishing the child.

Xuhuang's observations about the trauma of the surgery in her own body informed her decision to use infant formula. Seeking to navigate competing demands on her body required balancing her infant's needs while taking care of her own physical well-being. Infant formula provided the means to achieve this balance. In both these cases, we can also see the importance of women's relationships with mothers and mothers-in-law who supported their decisions to try alternatives to breastfeeding. Interestingly, Lu Bin overrode her mother-in-law's authority because she perceived formula to be safer, and therefore more beneficial, for the child. In these instances, we see the role that the experience and support of female kin may play in decisions about breast or bottle-feeding. These findings resonate with studies on the influence of older women's support on new mothers and infant feeding practices. Judy Aubel's review of infant feeding research and programs in the global south substantiates the need for more culturally relevant programs. She finds that the role of grandmothers throughout the global south may be central to new mothers' infant feeding decisions (2012).[8] A study from Nepal shows that grandmothers view themselves as central to the decision making and support of their daughter's infant feeding practices (Masvie 2006). Such findings suggest that infant feeding is a practice embedded in relationships that include kin as well as the mother and infant. Navigating situations like those that Lu Bin and Xuhuang found themselves in reinforces the conclusion that infant feeding decisions reflect logic and relations extending beyond those of the mother and child.

Lu Bin and Xuhuang were not alone in determining that they were producing insufficient milk for their newborns. Insufficient milk is one of the most common reasons around the world that women either mix breast and formula feeding or switch to exclusive formula feeding.[9] Women's observations that their milk was insufficient to satisfy their newborns have long concerned public health researchers and policy makers seeking to promote breastfeeding.[10] While scientific studies indicate that most women do have enough breast milk to nourish their children, it seems that little can be done to reassure mothers that this is the case. Anthropologists continue to contribute cross-cultural research findings so as to better understand such a common and pervasive explanation.[11] Research indicating that social learning may better predict women's infant feeding decisions reinforces my observation that the educational materials of the BFHI provided models of content or sleeping breastfed infants, not crying ones (Mok et al. 2008). Coupled with their understandings of traditional Chinese medical models of bodily depletion after childbirth, Lu Bin and Xuhuang's behavior becomes understandable.

Women found many ways to navigate around their mothers' and mothers-in-law's advice about how to feed their newborns. Some relied on support and advice from their husbands, while others invoked authoritative scientific and medical knowledge. Four months after the birth of her child, Lin Xianping, a twenty-four-year-old schoolteacher, discussed her decision to use western infant formula rather than a Chinese product.

> I use a foreign infant formula to feed my baby. It is from Holland. I decided to use infant formula (*naifen*) after one month of breastfeeding. I was sick with a cold and couldn't take any medicine for it because it would influence my breast milk. If I took the medicine, I couldn't feed my baby. Finally my doctor told me I needed to take some medicine, so I did, but then I couldn't use my milk to feed the baby. I had no choice. I talked to my husband and a friend who is a doctor.
>
> I didn't know whether to use Chinese or foreign formula. I think feeding an infant is the most important aspect of raising a child, so when I talked to my husband, he said that we must use the best substitute we could and that foreigners had been feeding their infants with formula for a long time and they had a more scientific culture than China's. Even though it costs us 200 to 300

> renminbi [yuan, approximately 40 to 50 US dollars] every month, I think it is worth it.
>
> My mother-in-law disagrees and thinks we can use cow's milk to feed the baby. She says she raised two children with cow's milk, and they were healthy. She also told me that you can't replace human milk anyway. She didn't support me, you know. But my doctor friend told me that foreign formula has many more nutrients than Chinese brands. Ordinary people, they think that cow's milk is good for infants; they think it should be fresh and [that] fresh milk is more nutritious. They think it can, at times, be better than the mother's breast milk, but they are ignorant. Foreign infant formula is most similar to breast milk. It is the most suitable for babies. Even though we spend more money, it is best for our child's health. This is most important.

Lin Xianping's narrative raises a number of issues related to good mothering, the authority of science, and consumerism. First, she links the product's safety to its western origins and calls on tradition—not the Chinese tradition, but the Western scientific tradition—to legitimize her choice. Moreover, to garner support for her decision, she sought the advice of a friend who was a medical doctor, a voice of authority. Additionally, as an educated consumer in China, she knows that local products might be unsafe or of unequal quality. Finally, she explicitly tells us how much money she spends on formula. Given that the couple's combined income ranged from 1,100 to 1,400 yuan per month, infant formula alone took up approximately 18 percent of their monthly income. Lin Xianping says that she can afford to buy foreign formula and in doing so is acting in a more modern manner than do those who use fresh cow's milk or Chinese infant formula to feed their infants. The symbols of science are embodied in the role of her doctor friend, whose medical authority is invoked when she describes her decision to go against the "ignorant" thinking of her mother-in-law. Finally, like the two women discussed above, Xianping privileges medical knowledge, as well as foreign scientific knowledge, over older female kin's experiential knowledge.

Lin Xianping's narrative reveals how she negotiated her role with her mother-in-law as well. As she contradicted her mother-in-law's experience with cow's milk and made her own decisions about how to best feed her baby, she asserted her authority as the child's mother. And yet the fact that she extensively researched infant formulas and gained the support of her doctor friend seems to indicate that the power of her mother-in-law was so strong that Xianping needed to arm herself with various types of external authority to make this decision. Furthermore, she reminded us and herself that the important thing was ultimately the child's health, and she articulated her decision to use foreign formula, rather than a Chinese brand, cow's milk, or breast milk in the context of this goal. Xianping's narrative demonstrates how the internalization of messages about the value of science, rather than tradition or experience, along with mobilization of resources outside the immediate family, come to shape decision making about the appropriate care of the single child. It is in such moments that we can see the process by which the agents of maternal governance shift from kin to science.

Zhai Xiurong, a twenty-five-year-old factory manager expressed similar sentiments. She started using infant formula as soon as she returned home from the hospital. Her mother stayed with her during the first month after the birth and helped her take care of her newborn while Zhai Xiurong was "doing the month." Like Lin Xianping, Zhai Xiurong rejected the traditions of her mother's generation as backward (*luohou de*) and antithetical to her desire to raise her son in the most modern, scientific way possible.

> I started using infant formula as soon as I returned home from the hospital. I attended the classes on breastfeeding at the hospital, but I knew that I would be returning to work, so I researched the infant formulas on the market and compared them. The Chinese products did not have as many nutrients as the foreign ones. I also asked my friends what formulas they had used. They mostly used foreign products as well. I thought if my baby can't have my milk he should have the most nutritious substitute I could buy.
>
> My mother wanted me to breastfeed. She had breastfed me and my sister and believes it is the best for infants, especially when

> they are very young. I told her that my work was important and I could not see trying to breastfeed for a few weeks and then having to switch to formula. It would be best for me and the baby if he got used to the formula right away. I also wanted to raise my son in the most modern, scientific way.
>
> China is developing quickly and becoming more modern; I want my son to benefit from these advances. The traditional ways are not good. I will take my son to a nursery school run by a woman who used to work as a psychologist. It is expensive and means I have to work more, but I don't want my mother or my mother-in-law raising my son using traditional methods. The foreign brand of infant formula is expensive, but I don't believe the Chinese formula companies are reliable; who controls them? The foreign companies have international standards that they have developed and they are more scientific. So I feel the foreign products are safer and provide better nutrition. Some of them even have more nutrients than breast milk!

Zhai Xiurong, like Lin Xianping, identifies foreign formula with modernity and science. She goes beyond feeding issues, however, by planning to enroll her son in a school run by a psychologist. Her strategies to avoid what she defines as "traditional" practices of child rearing will help prepare her son to operate in a competitive, global society.[12] Xiurong, by choosing to use scientific child-rearing methods and having her son literally consume the products of science and modernity through infant formula, echoes larger concerns with the local as inadequate. Rather than relying on government measures designed to protect consumers from low-quality or fake products and choosing to use one manufactured by a foreign entity, she believes she can ensure her son's well-being. She is not simply a new consumer but a globally aware one. Furthermore, her decisions and justifications for them reflect an individualized response to larger social issues no longer well controlled by the state. Whether her reasoning embodies a critique of the state's ability to manage itself is still unclear.

Other women could not, for many reasons, indulge in foreign

products. Cui Zhuhong, a twenty-seven-year-old office manager, also made the decision to switch to infant formula. She breastfed her daughter for six weeks and then gradually weaned her onto formula.

> I think that if a baby is healthy and has been breastfed during the first month after birth, it is all right to give it formula. After "doing the month," I felt that I had not lost the weight I had gained during pregnancy, and breastfeeding makes it difficult to lose weight. I just felt too fat and I knew I could not diet while breastfeeding, so after six weeks I stopped. My husband also told me that we could not have a sex life while I was breastfeeding. He felt that the breastfeeding was too depleting for my body and that sex would also be too much for me. I think he just thought that breastfeeding was a bit messy and it made him uncomfortable. I thought that if I could lose some weight, I would feel better too. Breastfeeding did make me feel tired a lot! So I stopped, and now I feel much better. My daughter is very healthy, and now that I am not breastfeeding my mother takes care of her during the day. It is just more convenient. It has been three months since I gave birth and my husband and I have a sex life, but now, after the baby, we are both so tired that it is not often that we have sex.

Cui Zhuhong's concerns reflect a different perspective from those of the previous narratives. She, too, is balancing competing pressures in her life, but the issue of her sexual relationship with her husband and her belief that she is overweight and will not be able to lose the weight while breastfeeding prompt her to stop. Moreover, she notes that her mother can care for her daughter because she is no longer breastfeeding and thus is less tied to the child. Interestingly, she does not mention work as a significant factor as she weighs her options. Rather, intimate relationships and the work of child rearing, as well as the desire to regain a prepregnancy bodily state, affected Cui Zhuhong's decision to use infant formula. Zhuhong's choices reflect the fact that the mid-1990s marked a pivotal shift in feminine ideals, bringing slimness and sexual availability to the forefront of some women's concerns.

In these cases, we see women negotiating with their older female kin as they accommodate the requirements of work, health, and marriage by deciding to switch to infant formula. They find this decision necessary because their bodily functions and shape do not conform to the demands of these contexts. These narratives also remind us that bodies are not simply the texts on which culture inscribes itself, but rather bodies and bodily functions are physiological and social entities (Turner 1994, 44).[13] Women who decide to use infant formula may be determining that the bodies of their infants can be well enough served with a breast milk substitute while their own bodies would be better off without the demands of breastfeeding.

Working and Infant Feeding

The issue of navigating the return to work and infant feeding was raised by Nurse Bai one day when we were talking about what things were like for women in the days before the economic reforms.

> We had no choice; there was little formula for our infants. Either you breastfed, or you tried to make do with cow's milk. But our jobs were arranged so that we could breastfeed. For me cow's milk was too expensive, so I took a nursing break every day and rode our family bicycle home to feed my son. It was a half-hour ride each way! But, the hospital gave me the time: my boss was a woman, and she gave me two hours so I could go home. It was very tiring though. I would ride home, feed the baby, eat, feed the baby again, clean up, and ride back to work. I rode my bicycle two hours every day for six months.
>
> Today women have choices; they can buy infant formula that is almost as good as their own milk. For working women, sometimes this is the only way they can stay in their jobs and feed their babies. Many places do not want to give women nursing breaks and people are living farther and farther away from their workplace, so they can't go home even if they want to. Work units do not want to spend money on nurseries for infants, and mothers might not

> want to put their children in the nursery because the quality of the caretakers might not be very good.

Nurse Bai's comments provide a context for the ways that women in my study responded to the multiple demands placed on them as they added the role of motherhood to their lives. They also exemplify the ironic situation: the economic reforms have brought about real changes in the availability of consumer goods that make life more convenient,[14] but at the same time, unlike the days when Nurse Bai was able to take extended (albeit strenuous) nursing breaks during her shift at the hospital, the economic reforms have created a workplace where women receive little institutional support for their roles as mothers.

Seven women in my sample continued to breastfeed up to four months (the state's recommended interval) and reported that they felt they were being good mothers by doing so. In some instances, workplace flexibility contributed to these women's ability to continue to breastfeed. Wang Yiqun, a twenty-four-year-old seamstress, said, "To be a good mother, I must give my son the best I can. Breastfeeding is the only way to protect and nurture him. If I didn't care about my child, I would just give him a bottle." The sentiment that a good mother breastfeeds her infant was echoed by other women, even when breastfeeding became difficult because of tension between maternal duties and work, as Feng Dongxin, a thirty-three-year-old manager in a state-owned company, told me.

> Breastfeeding is the best nutrition for my son, but it is also inconvenient for women who work outside the home. I can come home at lunch to feed my son because my office is close to my home, but it is still inconvenient at times for me to leave work. I have decided to have my cousin [who is taking care of the child] start giving him a bottle at lunchtime because, even though breast milk is best, I don't think it will influence his health too much if he drinks some formula. The other problem is that I have had a lot of milk, and it leaked in the first month of my return to work. I work in an office with men, and it is embarrassing to have this happen. I put pads

> and cloth in my bra, but sometimes I must carry an extra shirt or sweater to wear over my stained clothes. I don't like this at all. My son is almost four months old, and when he is about four months I am going to stop breastfeeding him. It is important to breastfeed infants, but after four months it is time to start adding foods, so it will be a good time to start using formula too. Then I can stop worrying about my milk leaking when I am at work!

Feng Dongxin believed that breastfeeding was best for her baby, but it required that she negotiate it with the demands of the workplace, where her maternal body did not conform to her professional image. For her child, whose nurturance depended on her physical presence, relying on a female family member, who was not an authority figure and thus tractable, to bottle-feed the child during work hours was a solution.[15]

Chang Guixing, a twenty-seven-year-old worker in a clothing factory, opted to take a longer maternity leave than most of the women in this study because she wanted to breastfeed her infant for four months.

> Breastfeeding is so important for the baby's health. My factory offered me a year's maternity leave, but I felt that I should only take four months. This is the recommended time for breastfeeding. The factory offers women long leaves so they don't have to pay them bonuses and other extra money. One woman told me that when she was pregnant, the factory leaders offered her a two-year maternity leave at 50 percent of her salary. She decided not to do this because her family could not afford it. I took four months because we could afford it and because I thought it was important to stay home while the baby is so small. I am glad I have stayed home during this time. I think my baby's health is most important. My work will still be there when I return. If I took a year, it might be hard for my family. We would not have enough money. But if I had to buy formula, that costs money too.

Chang Guixing's decision to take a longer maternity leave than most women in this study was not the norm. Though entitled to at least ninety days' leave with pay, the majority of women (twenty-eight out of thirty) only took eight- to ten-week maternity leaves. Guixing calculated that the extra time away from her job would not have an overly negative effect on either the family finances or her position when she returned to work. But while her decisions and actions differed from those of other women I have described, she, too, made decisions that ultimately reflected the ways in which some workplaces tried to support the competing demands of mothering and work. But Chang Guixing's decision to stay home also indicates that workplace accommodations ultimately could not help her if she wished to complete the prescribed four months of breastfeeding and so it was she who would have to sacrifice to stay home.[16]

Che Yan's description of negotiating breastfeeding while she worked at her family's business indicates that her flexible working conditions allowed her to care for her child.

> I am still breastfeeding [at four months] because it is the best, most natural way to nourish my infant. He is a strong, healthy baby—he is rarely sick, and I believe that my milk protects him. I returned to work after taking a two-month leave, but our home is right behind the printshop; I just move back and forth with the baby. While he sleeps, I work out front, and when I need to feed him I just go in back and get him. If we are busy, my mother comes and stays with us. Otherwise, it has been very easy for me to breastfeed.

Not all women engaged in a family business could afford the luxuries Che Yan enjoyed. One woman who ran a small tailoring business with her husband tried, with his help, to care for her daughter, but after four months they felt the business was suffering. The couple made a decision they described as "painful" to send the child to their family in Sichuan.

For some women, difficulties with breastfeeding did not result in a switch to infant formula even when working outside the home. Ke Hong, a twenty-six-year-old department store worker, described her trials and tenacity in the early days of trying to breastfeed her daughter one day after the infant's checkup in the hospital.

> Breastfeeding is difficult! No one told me that my nipples would be sore, my breasts hurt, or that it would make me feel so tired. In the hospital, I had some problems holding the baby so that she suckled properly and it was so painful. The nurse or my mother would tell me that I should try feeding my daughter, and I would just think about the pain and not want to do it. Sometimes when I breastfed her in those first days I just cried because my whole body was in pain and I felt so weak.
>
> When I returned home, the situation did not improve for a long time. My breasts became engorged with milk, and the baby could not drink enough to help relieve the pain. I had to use my hands to get the milk out. It was so much trouble! All I did was eat, sleep, feed the baby, and squeeze milk out of my breasts. I was not very happy at the time. After about two months, everything seemed easier. I think I regained my strength, the baby started sleeping better, I learned [from my mother] how to breastfeed so that it was not so painful, and everything became more peaceful in my life.
>
> Now [at five months] everything is fine. I am glad that I continued to breastfeed because my daughter is very healthy and content. My mother helped me a lot in the first two months. She encouraged me a lot even when I lost my temper or cried. Now I feel that I have done the best I could for my daughter. I only breastfeed twice a day now because she is starting to eat food and soon I will wean her, maybe at six months.
>
> It has not always been convenient to breastfeed. The difficulties at the beginning are one aspect of this. But, when I went back to work after three months of maternity leave, it was also a problem for me. I do not live far from my workplace, but sometimes my milk would start to come in before I could get home to feed my daughter. I just had to wash a lot of clothes at that time.

Here Ke Hong's mother became the ultimate teacher about breastfeeding, despite her stay in the BFH. Ke Hong manages the bodily and logistical challenges of breastfeeding at work in part because of the convenience of living close to her workplace. More recent research shows that work continues to play an important role in women's sense of self and that white-collar women workers in cities like Shanghai, often referred to as "white-collar beauties" (*bailing liren*), seek ways to balance motherhood and work as they care for their infants. Sun Zhongxin's study of middle-class mothers in Shanghai shows that education, financial independence, and employment in foreign companies can provide women with the means to maintain their professional and maternal identities (2008). These women found that at a foreign company their gender and reproductive potential played only a small role in their work. Rather, women believed that they were judged on their performance. Whether they retired temporarily from the workforce to raise their children or continued to work and relied on paid help from nannies and housekeepers, the women in Sun's study found satisfaction in both aspects of their identities.

The pressures of employment, especially for those women in my study who returned to work after a two- to three-month maternity leave, shaped infant feeding decisions. Many who had been breastfeeding stopped and transitioned their children to infant formula so that others could care for them (Sun 2008, 25). Women's decisions remain very personal, individual, and in large part unpredictable. Women in this study who worked close to home did have some advantages but not enough to tip the balance between breast and bottle-feeding. Mothers and mothers-in-law could become important supporters of breastfeeding or advocates of alternatives. What we learn is that women do have choices within certain constraints and that they navigate among their options as best they can to satisfy myriad expectations. In their creatively pragmatic actions, two factors remain constant—the desire to work and the desire to maintain a modicum of independence from those family members whose interventions might or might not be welcome. Finally, these women's decisions and choices as mothers and workers provide microlevel insight into recent studies in China showing that, despite increased income stratification and differences in women's and men's pursuit of employment, both high- and low-income families maintain traditional gendered divisions of labor—child rearing remains the domain of women (Kim Won et al. 2010, 957).[17]

Child Rearing and Modernity

In the same vein, issues of child care for these women brought up changing ideas about the modern and the traditional. When women were "doing the month," the opposition between notions of modernity and tradition were formulated by all parties around certain assumptions about hygiene and food. As the women and their husbands decided how to set their only children on the path to their best development, the old ways and modern trends again became important in their narratives. In almost all cases, the young couples in Beijing believed that their parents' beliefs about child rearing were backward and unscientific. The narratives presented here offer interesting insights into the dynamics of resistance and accommodation and the impact of status and household economics. If women could afford a *bao mu* (children's nurse), they hired a woman who would live with them and care for their children. Most women, however, could not afford this option either because of limited space or finances or because they already lived with their mothers-in-law or mothers. Twenty-one women told me that their mothers or mothers-in-law were caring for their children. Women's mothers or their husbands' mothers often became default caretakers because of such living arrangements, but this was not considered ideal by the majority of my sample.

Perceptions of the ideal child care situation varied. Some women thought that a day care facility was a good option for developing a child's mental skills, while others wanted to hire a *bao mu* who could pay sole attention to their children.[18] Nannies often came from places like Anhui Province and other relatively remote regions of China. Beijing residents often denigrate these women as backward and undeveloped. Furthermore these young rural women are generally not well educated or trained in any particular skills that would suit them for child rearing. Yet, as Li Yurong, a twenty-four-year-old office worker, said:

> If we had enough money, I would hire a *bao mu* to care for my daughter. Right now my mother is caring for her. She lives close to

> us, and it is free and convenient. But I think her ideas about child rearing are old-fashioned, and she spoils my daughter!

When asked why a nanny would make a better caretaker, given that these women are often from rural areas and do not have much education, she replied:

> You are right, they are not well educated and are not wordly (*meiyou wenhua*), but they are working for you. With my mother, I see her spoiling my daughter, and it is hard to criticize her way of doing things. I am not paying her, and she is my mother! With a *bao mu,* you are able to supervise (*guan li*) them, and this means that you can use more modern, scientific methods to raise your child. With my mother, I can't tell her how to do anything; she has already raised me, and so she thinks she knows how to raise my daughter. But right now we don't have the money.

Li Yurong's comments raise the issue of power: she saw her mother's set beliefs as too hard to change, and, unlike differences of opinion over infant feeding methods, the day-to-day decisions about child rearing could not become a battleground without cost to the family. Only in a contractual relationship or an agreement with a less authoritative female kinswoman could the young mother exert her individual plan for raising a modern child. The issue, then, was not simply one of "tradition" over "modernity" but one of individual control and the young mother's confidence in her understanding of the modern world's demands. Furthermore, the purchase of another's labor would bring a new set of consumer relations into the mix. I must mention here, however, that having helpful relatives close at hand might seem like a luxury to unfortunate couples like the tailors, who had to send their child to a distant province to be reared without any input from them.

Women who could not afford a *bao mu* or day care facility still found ways to bypass the problem of having a mother or mother-in-law care for their children. Wu Qiuping, a twenty-five-year-old worker, found a young female cousin from the countryside who could live with her and her husband and care for their child. Wu Qiuping's mother-in-law lived near them and helped out, but Qiuping did not want her to raise their son. Her cousin, she said, was happy to be living in the city (albeit illegally), and she listened to Wu Qiuping about taking care of the baby. They paid her a small salary, some pocket money, and her expenses. Qiuping said that their apartment was small, so the young woman slept in the living room on a foldout couch. She was comfortable with this arrangement because, she said, "she is my cousin; she is family." Once again we see that one way for a new mother to maintain control of the direction and nature of her child's care and education was to avoid the less desirable arrangement of having an older woman care for the child.

In these cases, we see women actively seeking ways to take control of their children's care while they continued to work. Such instances demonstrate that women must make a number of accommodations in the ways they care for their children, whether it be decisions about breast or formula feeding, or the choice of caretaker, and attempt to maintain their authority and presence in caring for their only child. Moreover, these examples indicate that for many the ideal of a modern, scientific method of child rearing is more desirable than the methods used by their more traditional parents and older family members.

The meanings these women assigned to old-fashioned child-rearing practices were fairly uniform, centering on worries about spoiling and lack of discipline. But what modernity meant to them was more difficult to elicit. To Zhang Yaoxing it meant that children should not be spoiled, that they should learn to listen to adults, and that they needed to be taught things such as drawing, music, and exercise. To Yang Huizhi, a twenty-six-year-old factory worker, it meant that after the age six months children needed to be stimulated by having stories read to them and by receiving help in learning to play with toys. They should not be beaten or hit for almost any reason. She also said:

> I was not raised using modern methods. At that time [end of the Cultural Revolution], my sister and I were often left alone with

> our neighbor, an older woman. I was five, and my sister was two years old, and we did not really do much but play outside, eat, and sleep. I remember being hit several times when I did not come home for dinner because I wanted to stay outside. I don't think children should be hit for any reason. Especially young children, they do not understand anything, and if you hit them, they just remember that, not why you hit them.

Physical punishment no longer seemed appropriate, but discipline inculcated from a young age was important for success in an increasingly competitive world. Mental stimulation was also given attention, as Zhou Xiuying states.

> I want my son to have the best education possible, and this means that even at a young age his mind and body must be stimulated and strengthened. As his mother, I feel that I can help keep him healthy by feeding him nutritious foods. I can help him develop good skills and intelligence and help him to study hard when he goes to school. But even now when he is only one year old, I think he needs to have his mind stimulated. So I read books to him and help him play with things that increase his dexterity (*ling huo de*).

In this case and the others presented above, clearly the state's aim to produce a modern, healthy population of future citizens was one shared by these mothers. However, their motivations to help their children develop and grow in the most scientific and modern ways available may also indicate that these parents were less than certain about the future. The state's program of economic reform had certainly improved urban living standards in ways that were unimaginable in the past, but these improvements had come with some costs. In particular, little job security existed for even the most successful young people. The socialist market economy had brought the concept and reality of capitalist forms of competition into people's consciousness as more and more state-owned enterprises were being weaned from the purse strings of a centralized government and individuals were finding that their iron-rice-bowl jobs no longer guaranteed work. These changes were clearly influencing the way these mothers anticipated and planned for their children's future. They believed that they needed to raise children who could participate in a system in which independence and entrepreneurial initiative were most likely to lead to financial success and security.[19]

The one-child policy plays an important role in this process as well. Parents have one child on which to focus their energies and aspirations, and this intense focus on the child has brought the issue of parenting into the realm of science and modernity in ways that are new to socialist China. For example, a new trend in the 1990s was sending couples to "parents school" so they could learn better, more modern parenting skills and educate their children using psychological tools and scientific methods. (Zhu 2010). The advent of these schools may have been an attempt by the state to intervene in the process of child rearing in order to mitigate the individualism that had been creeping into the consciousness of its citizenry since the reforms (Ong 1997). These schools may also have been intended to shape future citizens at the earliest stages of their development by inculcating in their parents values that would help create a more modern population. The pressures women in this study felt portended the future. In the intervening years, the popularity of a 2013 reality television show called Where Are We Going, Dad?, which followed celebrity fathers as they interacted with their children, indicates that in the twenty-first century parents still seek sources of information on how best to raise their children. One young mother watched the show in order to reflect on her parenting practices. She noted, "Not only can you see the spirit of young parents, but also you can relate yourself to the characters." (Zhu 2014). Teresa Kuan documents the moral dilemmas faced by middle-class parents in twenty-first-century China's modernization project. She shows that they must navigate new expectations about parenting to balance the psychological well-being of their child at a time when competition has permeated all realms of society and the possibilities for getting a good education and achieving economic success are scarce (2015).

The aspirations of modernity in the 1990s, whether expressed by the state or the mothers in my study, were still being mediated by extended family relations in terms of child rearing. Not only did mothers and mothers-in-law most often serve as the primary caretakers for the young children of these women, but economically the larger family networks were important to the child's well-being. The average income of the women in my study was about 800 to 1,100 yuan per month (approximately 89 to 112 US dollars). This was well above the average for the country. Women told me that their families contributed both money and goods to help raise their children. The amount varied, but all women said that both sets of parents regularly contributed money, food, clothing, and toys to their immediate households. This parental economic assistance may have affected some of the independence the women sought as they made decisions about how to raise their children. Bi Hongxia, a twenty-six-year-old woman who worked in a small family-owned (her husband's) factory, told me that when she decided to switch to infant formula her mother-in-law offered to help pay for the more expensive foreign brand that she wanted to give her child.

> When my milk was not enough for the baby, the doctor told me to start adding some infant formula. When I asked other women what formula to use, they all suggested that I use a foreign brand because they are higher quality products. But they are also very expensive compared to the Chinese brands. My mother-in-law told me that she would help pay for the foreign formula since it is better. We spend between 300 and 400 renminbi [yuan] on infant formula every month, and my mother-in-law gives me between 200 and 400 to help pay for it.

While Bi Hongxia did not mention that she had any differences with her mother-in-law over how to raise her daughter, she did say that in many ways her mother-in-law was traditional, especially about "doing the month." However, such economic ties could come into play over major decisions about how to care for the child. I asked women whether they felt that economic ties between them and their parents had any influence on the decisions they made about their children. None of them thought this was true, but they all believed that when it came time to send the child to nursery school or kindergarten their parents might impose their own views. Otherwise, they said, they could not think of instances in which the money or goods had any major effect on their decisions.

Women who can afford the time and money to invest in their children today do so for the same reasons women in China have always chosen: a child represents security in old age. But the task has become more complex in the reform era. Filial piety, respect for elders, and even a capacity for learning are not sufficient to ensure the economic success of a household in urban China today. Mental agility and good health also become important, and women who can afford it invest in promoting these traits in their children.[20] But at the same time they try to find ways to assert their own control over the process, just as in the 1990s they figured out strategies for feeding their infants that moved between elders and tradition and familial obligations and their own desires for independence.

Conclusion

Since the mid-1990s the tensions that women face between home and work have continued to assert themselves in popular and state contexts. In 2001 Wang Xiancai, a National Committee member of the Chinese People's Consultative Conference, presented a proposal to encourage married working women to leave their jobs and become housewives in order to alleviate unemployment and improve family life (*Beijing Review,* April 25, 2001).[21] The proposal inspired debate among the members, whose discussions revealed that China's government was using the very real issues of women's double burden as mothers and workers, the high costs of child care, and the increasingly valued position of home life as an escape from public life to alleviate its own problems. Interestingly, Wang suggested that Chinese society could more closely emulate more developed countries where, he observed, "The couples divide family responsibilities, with many women leaving their jobs after childbirth to raise children"

(*Beijing Review,* April 25, 2001). Associating his proposal with modern, developed economies certainly plays on broader popular and official concerns that China must rapidly and purposefully catch up to these countries. Wang's proposal underscores the fact that the very real difficulties facing working mothers in this study continue in the twenty-first century.

Encouraging women to become housewives and mothers is not a new solution for the Chinese state.[22] Resolving unemployment by returning women to home and family, as proposed by the central government official, however, relies on individual rather than institutional solutions to a social problem. The gendered nature of such a proposal might be better understood as the manifestation of what Evans calls the "feminization of intimacy," embodying both state and individual interests, needs, and desires (Evans 2010, 981). She finds that the feminization of intimacy arises out of the intersection of broader processes of naturalizing women's roles, reinforced by the state in popular discourse and women's precarious position in the job market, and changes in individual women's hopes for intimacy in their family relationships. Decisions about how women balance work and nourish infants help demonstrate the workings of the feminization of intimacy.[23]

Finally, new solutions to the problem of providing Chinese infants with breast milk made international news in 2006 when it was reported that rural women were taking jobs as wet nurses in urban Shenzhen and Beijing. High salaries promised to these women made such positions attractive since a babysitter typically makes between three and eight hundred renminbi per month and wet nurses are garnering monthly salaries of up to eight thousand. Wet nursing has a long tradition in China, but it is associated with the past and thus has sparked controversy about whether such work is exploitative (Kwan 2006). The resurgence of wet nursing in China should not come as a surprise given that Chinese women, like those in this study, have found themselves negotiating among competing pressures at work and in the family; an increasingly consumer-oriented society that emphasizes choice, individuality, desire, and competition; and the imperatives of the state's reproductive health policies. An unanticipated but creative solution for some women who seek to resolve such pressures, wet nursing embodies the contradictions of market socialism. Its resurgence further reinforces the necessity of understanding how outcomes of health decisions, such as whether to breastfeed or not, result from complex, contextual, and/or individual situations.

Conclusion

> A miracle substance that reduces ear infections while seeming to raise scores on I.Q. tests by several points? Available even in the most remote villages, requiring no electricity or refrigeration? Oh, and as long as we're dreaming, let's make it free. . . . Sometimes the solutions are dazzlingly high-tech, but almost nothing could save as many children's lives each year as nature's own miracle: breast milk.
>
> —Nicholas Kristoff

As Nicholas Kristoff's plea to women across the globe (*New York Times,* October 22, 2015), even those far from urban centers, indicates, the mystery and wonder of breast milk is universal and timeless. As this book has shown, the benefits of breast milk have been endorsed by science and yet are believed to be transmitted to infants without human intervention. The conviction that breastfeeding is a "free" low-tech solution that can save the world's children persists in the twenty-first century and may come as no surprise to readers. Indeed, Kristoff's dictum reinforces the notion of the potential of breast milk and breastfeeding to shape the future by saving infants from death, and under less dire circumstances, by producing healthy, intelligent children. The biological and social messages intertwined in such views produce an almost absolute moral case for breastfeeding. Why would one turn down "free" breast milk, with biological properties so powerful that they can prevent ear infections and build stronger immune systems?

This book has looked at what happens when such assumptions and logics of potentiality about breastfeeding enter into the spaces of a hospital and transmit to urban Chinese women messages about how to feed their only children. It has drawn attention to the converging constellation of relations and power in the BFH—from global health policies to consumer culture, national economic and demographic agendas, family relations, and gender ideals—that women must navigate as they become mothers. These external demands created constraints and opportunities within which individual women maneuvered as they made decisions about how to best care for their infants and maintain their sense of self. It should be clear that there was no single formula for becoming a mother and making infant feeding decisions in the period covered here.

We have also seen how the changes that occurred during the mid-1990s in China reinforce the importance of examining global health projects in broader political and economic contexts and as forms of maternal governance. In the case of China, the government sought (as it continues to seek) to increase its power and presence on the international political scene, maintain internal political control and national stability, and yet allow for the individual economic choices on which a market economy based on consumer desires depends. The manifestations of these state agendas in women's lives have been shown to vary in relation to reproductive timelines. During pregnancy, women hear the message that the state's interest in child health is paramount as it creates BFHs throughout urban China. Such efforts have brought China recognition as a world leader in breastfeeding promotion because they address a public health concern long on the agendas of the WHO and UNICEF. During their recoveries and return to work, women are balancing the imperatives of feeding their infants with their work and family obligations as more direct interventions to promote breastfeeding recede.

The reach of China's BFHI also suggests significant success in promoting breastfeeding. According to a report compiled by the National Health and Family Planning Commission, in 2015 China continued to lead the world with more than seven thousand baby-friendly-certified hospitals (Liu 2016). Of all Chinese births in 2014, 66 percent occurred in these hospitals and 92 percent of infants were exclusively breastfed while in the hospital (Liu 2016). Early research points to success outside the hospital as well: exclusive breastfeeding rates in rural areas rose from 29 percent in 1992 to 68 percent in 1994, and in urban areas the increase was from 10 to 48 percent (UNICEF 2005). More recent studies of breastfeeding's prevalence in China present a mixed picture. A study of Jinan City in 2000 showed that 35 percent of infants under four months were exclusively breastfed (Zhao et al. 2003). Results from a 2004–5 prospective study of 1,520 women in Zhejiang Province found that less than 5 percent of infants were exclusively breastfed for six months and 98 percent consumed infant formula at some point in their first six months. Factors affecting women's decisions to mix breastfeeding with infant formula or switch exclusively to infant formula among the women in this study included returning to work within six months of childbirth, urban residence, and the early introduction of liquids (Qiu et al. 2010). These mixed results resonate with the experiences of women in other countries that have undertaken the BFHI and serve as a reminder of the complexity of infant feeding decisions and practices.

In the aftermath of the 2008 melamine-tainted formula scandal the Chinese government renewed its commitment to promoting breastfeeding as part of the National Basic Public Health Service Program, and studies since then have continued to exhibit patterns similar to earlier findings. For example, Zhenyu Yang and her colleagues, in a 2013 study of 14,530 children from fifty-five counties in thirty provinces, showed that about 20 percent of infants were breastfeeding at six months (2016). Research in poor counties in western China found that about 28 percent of infants under six months had been exclusively breastfed (Guo et al. 2013). By contrast, a study in Hunan presented a more optimistic picture in which researchers found that 45 percent of infants had been exclusively breastfed for six months

(Qin et al. 2017). Such wide-ranging findings may be the result of several factors, including definitions of exclusive breastfeeding, study design, and research methodology. Information about the women we have followed in this book, from their musings about pregnancy to their lives as working mothers, provides a crucial addition to these large-scale studies of infant feeding practices. The longitudinal and ethnographic perspective taken here helps to contextualize the mixed results of China's breastfeeding promotion efforts by bringing our attention to the agents of maternal governance at work in women's lives and the creative ways in which they balance their infants' well-being with other demands. Together they show us that infant feeding decisions are complex.

Perhaps these women's strategies can also help us understand why, despite the risks associated with infant formula, especially after the melamine tainting of 2008, it continues to serve as an important source of nourishment for China's infants. Research studies among China's affluent families indicate that infant formula continues to be a popular adjunct to or substitute for breastfeeding. However, money and transnational social networks allow these privileged families to bypass potentially tainted Chinese formula by purchasing imported foreign brands. Hanser and Li (2015) draw on interview and popular media sources to show that these consumption practices appear to confirm how individualized consumer strategies can inhibit opportunities for collective action and demonstrate that "opting out" calls into question the state's legitimacy as a protector of its citizens. But for ordinary people outside or on the margins of China's large metropolitan centers such options may have little salience. The quantitative research bears this out: poorer women tend to breastfeed more and for longer durations than their wealthier counterparts do (Qiu et al. 2010).

The success in achieving high rates of breastfeeding within the BFH reinforces the usefulness of looking at these spaces through an anthropological lens. Focusing on the clinics and wards in a hospital provides a bounded space in which we can witness the way everyday practices and technologies of medicine come to support ideas about gender, bodies, reproduction, consumerism, globalization, and the nation in a rapidly changing social milieu. The convergence of these forces in the hospital, however, is also contingent on historical, political, and social circumstances. Exploring the daily workings of a Chinese hospital's obstetrics clinic and wards brings a more localized understanding of the way such circumstances shape and are shaped by the individuals who work and seek care there. While health practitioners like Nurse Bai certainly play a critical role in promoting and enacting broader agendas about maternal and child health, the shape of these actions depends on the life histories and circumstances that women bring to the hospital. Simultaneously embracing a global policy to increase breastfeeding and welcoming infant formula sales representatives and their products in the hospital become about more than the tension between collective and individual interests in new mothers' lives or even corruption. Rather, health professionals seek to mediate the imperatives of the state to resolve the contradictions they experience and witness in the hospital and more generally as citizens of the nation. As agents of maternal governance, they navigate the terrain of state policy and what is best for new mothers.[1]

While the hospital frames reproductive processes and dynamics in the pre- and postnatal periods, after the birth of a child, other institutional forces come to the fore in women's negotiations with motherhood. The spaces of the workplace organized in a market-based economy resulting from state policy agendas to modernize China have made it increasingly difficult for mothers to balance their work lives and the demands of motherhood. As increasing numbers of state and private enterprises seek to maximize profits, women's reproductive lives have come to symbolize an impediment to profit seeking in the workplace. The demands of the workplace and women's desire to continue their employment in this environment increasingly require women to individually strategize to manage motherhood and work. Maintaining these commitments is not necessarily new or unique to women in China or indeed the world. However, under socialism the problems of blending motherhood and work were perceived as requiring institutional rather than individual solutions.[2] Indeed, it is in the realm of the workplace that the retreat of state-level support for mothers since the 1980s is most apparent. However, the intrinsic value of wage labor to women's equality and autonomy as promoted during the Mao years continues to shape many women's belief that they can balance working and mothering. In addition to the economic necessity of maintaining employment, many of the mothers followed in this study viewed their work as part of their identity and a space where they found autonomy from the family.

Messages in the workplace and other spaces outside the hospital make clear the bodily demands facing women in the 1990s and the twenty-first century. Lactating bodies do not have a place in the work environment. Moreover, the prepregnant slim and increasingly sexualized body represents a crucial standard to which new mothers are held. Reconciling their bodily experiences with these representations and expectations took different forms for women in this study. Some sought to realign their bodies with the demands of the workplace by transitioning to bottle-feeding while others found ways to manage and balance the demands of work and breastfeeding. Such discourse reveals an expanded form of maternal governance that arises in indirect ways outside breastfeeding policies, and women's responses remind us that navigating multiple demands leads women to find a variety of ways to balance these demands.

The one-child policy also brings into relief the ways in which a strategy to reshape family structures in the interest of modernizing the nation defines the parameters within which individuals must negotiate. One of the overt forms of maternal governance in women's lives—limiting reproduction for the good of the nation—functions as an apparatus that concurrently restricts and creates possibilities for new mothers. On the one hand, the stakes are high for the mother of an only child for she must rear a healthy and intelligent son or daughter who will succeed in the uncertain economic milieu fostered by capitalism. Yet we see that from pregnancy to the early months of their children's lives mothers both create opportunities and accede to constraints as they navigate changeable social and economic landscapes.

An additional social force that shaped the context in which women became mothers in the 1990s was the emerging consumer culture in urban China. Although the hospital brought some aspects of consumerism to the fore, external expressions and definitions of beauty, sexuality, and femininity evident in advertising, popular magazines, television, and other media created yet another milieu requiring navigation. Reforming the reproductive body into one capable of work and sexual relations became another arena of women's lives requiring management and control. As individual women sought ways to cope with their desires, fears, and bodily manifestations, they demonstrated through their actions that such imperatives were key sites of struggle about the meaning and experience of gender and self in 1990s China.

Throughout this book, I have focused on the responses of thirty ordinary working women to institutionalized agendas, from global health policies to new expectations of femininity and beauty as a kind of creative pragmatism. The women in this study have shown us that as they made decisions at numerous junctures in the runup to motherhood, they did so in self-conscious ways that help us see how agency plays out in everyday practice. These women cannot be viewed simply as products of their social roles (Lock and Kaufert 2001; Mohanty 2003). The range of incidents that illustrate women's decisions, from leaving a breastfeeding class early because the information did not seem relevant to hiring an outsider to help with child care in order to avoid the outdated child-rearing practices of older kin, serves as a reminder that the seemingly insignificant, as well as the more obvious, actions of women contribute to a formation of a sense of self as a mother. Tradition and kinship demands present constraints in everyday life, as we saw in the practices of doing the month. Yet women found ways to manage the goal of producing a healthy child for their own benefit by navigating among these messages and traditions. We have seen that even within the hospital, health workers displayed much creativity in using a welter of seemingly meaningless messages to convey their own truths. And women who were entering new territory as they became mothers in a consumerist culture managed to pick and choose the products and practices that would best suit them.

The biological time of gestation and the concomitant bodily changes experienced by the women in this study show that their ideas, experiences, and actions related to motherhood were conditional and fluctuant. During pregnancy and childbirth, and to an extent in the early postpartum period, most did not find it essential to actively participate in all aspects of their care. While their behavior during these times indicates that they were active participants in some ways, as they recovered from birth many of them began to more forcefully define and put into action their desires for their children and themselves. Their actions, whether related to breastfeeding, choosing a form of child care, or dieting, became important to the process of defining the parameters of motherhood within multiple layers of constraints. It is in these decisions that women's creative pragmatism becomes most apparent and illustrates the variety of ways in which one can become a mother and nourish a child.

The lack of clear, categorized responses to the variety of imperatives that the mothers in this study faced, such as whether to breastfeed or not, shows that power relations are not easily represented as dualistic dynamics between state and citizen or conformity and dissent (Greenhalgh 2008; Lupton 1995, 3). What is possible, in the realms created by structures of power, are mothers who make constrained choices and decisions (Rose 2007).

Appendix 1

Table 1. Summary of Participants in Sample ($N = 30$)

Name	Age at Marriage	Age at Pregnancy	Occupation	Education Level	Coresidents	Mother's Origin	Mother-in-Law's Origin
Wu Qiuping	24	25	factory worker	middle school	in-laws	urban	rural
Zhai Xiurong	25	25	factory manager	middle school	parents	urban	urban
Zhu Xuhuang	24	24	factory worker	middle school	husband	urban	urban
Lin Xianping	24	24	teacher	college	in-laws	rural	urban
Feng Dongxin	28	33	administrator	technical school	parents	rural	rural
Zhang Yaoxin	24	24	secretary	high school	in-laws	urban	urban
Shen Jun	24	24	family business	middle school	husband	rural	rural
Qu wen	24	25	pharmacy tech	technical school	husband	rural	rural
Lu Bin	25	27	publications manager	technical school	in-laws	urban	urban
Gu Lijuan	25	26	administrator	technical school	in-laws	urban	urban
Xie Jinmei	22	22	factory worker	middle school	parents	urban	urban

Table 1.—*Continued*

Name	Age at Marriage	Age at Pregnancy	Occupation	Education Level	Coresidents	Mother's Origin	Mother-in-Law's Origin
Cui Zhuhong	25	27	office manager	high school	in-laws	urban	urban
Chen Yan	26	27	store manager	technical school	husband	urban	rural
Bi Hongxia	25	26	family business	middle school	husband	urban	rural
Che Yan	25	26	family business	middle school	husband	rural	rural
Du Yan	24	24	buyer	high school	in-laws	urban	urban
Wang Yiqun	24	24	family business	middle school	in-laws	rural	urban
Chang Guixiang	24	27	factory worker	middle school	in-laws	urban	urban
Li Yurong	24	24	office worker	technical school	in-laws	urban	urban
Yang Huzhi	23	23	store worker	primary school	parents	rural	urban
Sun Li Mei	28	30	factory worker	middle school	husband	urban	urban
Han Aihua	23	23	office worker	middle school	in-laws	urban	urban
Xi Jun	24	24	family business	primary school	husband	rural	rural
Bian Shuli	23	24	administrator	college	husband	urban	rural
Shi Binyan	27	31	engineer	university	husband	urban	urban
Ke Hong	24	26	store worker	middle school	in-laws	urban	urban
Yan Daifeng	27	29	printshop worker	middle school	husband	urban	urban
Zhou Xiuying	28	30	nurse	technical college	husband	rural	rural
Huang Fengyin	24	24	family business	middle school	in-laws	rural	rural
Yang Zhiyun	25	26	factory worker	middle school	parents	rural	urban

Notes

Introduction

1. On American BFHs, see http://www.babyfriendlyusa.org/find-facilities. India in 2002 had 1,250 (http://www.unicef.org/nutrition/index_24806.html).

2. Prior to the Communist Revolution in 1949, foreign infant formula was available in many large cities (see Glosser 1999). After 1949 it was not readily available. Substitutes such as cow's milk were used, although it was rationed due to its scarcity (Pasternak and Wang 1985).

3. This study builds on research about the intersection between government intervention in reproduction in China and other parts of the world and the strategies used by ordinary people to order their lives in their own interest. See, for example, Greenhalgh 2008; Rivkin-Fish 2005; Murphy 2012; Browner and Sargent 2011; Van Hollen 2003, 2011; Allen 2002; Paxson 2004; and Kanaaneh 2002.

4. The edited volume by Kipnis (2012) offers insights into the individualization occurring in twenty-first-century China and seeks to complicate our understandings of the individual and modernity. Kleinman et al. (2011) suggest that the balance between possibilities for individualism and state control create dissonance within the self. Yan (2009) demonstrates how individuals in post-Mao China found opportunities to break from the socialist institutions and practices of the recent past. Zhang and Ong (2007) show that liberal theorists' assumption that with economic liberalization comes political liberalization does not hold in China. Rather, they show that the

state simultaneously creates opportunities for individual differentiation and maintains absolute control in other ways and that this balance allows the Chinese Communist Party (CCP) to retain its power.

5. See, for example, Jelliffe and Jelliffe 1978; Dettwyler and Fishman 1992; Obermayer and Castle 1996; Huffman 1984; and Cattaneo 2012.

6. *Biopolitics* refers to a government's interest in managing the health and well-being of its population. Foucault was referring to national governments in his theory, but the extension to international units of governance like the WHO is changing the scale at which we seek to document biopolitics (Foucault 1990, 139; Rabinow and Rose 2006, 197). For an examination of biopolitics and China's one-child policy, see also Greenhalgh 2005; and Greenhalgh and Winkler 2005.

7. I have developed a theoretical framework (Greenhalgh 2008) that draws on government and scientific studies to parse this process in terms of China's birth-planning policy (the one-child policy).

8. Foucault called this aspect of biopower anatomo-politics (1990, 139). See also Allen 2002, 2–5, which describes the use of Mrs. X, a third world everywoman, in a lecture on maternal mortality by a senior medical officer of the WHO.

9. See McCaughey 2010 for insights drawn from personal experience and a feminist analysis of the complexity and challenges that breastfeeding may present.

10. The video can be viewed at https://www.youtube.com/watch?v=1F9Py-OlNdA.

11. See also Ottawa Charter for Public Health, Geneva, Switzerland, World Health Organization 1986. Awofeso (2004) provides an overview of the major shifts in public health work and questions whether the new public health is so new. Public health at earlier points in history worked alongside hospital- or clinic-based medicine at the population level as it served to control communicable diseases not by treating individuals but by quarantine and sanitation measures that minimized the spread of disease. Hospital medicine and its public health counterpart continue to play an important role in the health system, but since the early twentieth century they have been accompanied by the development of health promotion. See Armstrong 1995; Gastaldo 1997; and Lupton 1995.

12. See also the Innocenti Declaration (World Health Organization 1981), ratified by thirty-two governments (including China) in 1990, which calls for more support for global breastfeeding.

13. Ginsburg and Rapp's introduction to their edited volume (1995) brought this logic to anthropology's attention.

14. See Van Esterik 1989; Maher 1992; Wolf 2010; and Bartlett and Shaw 2010.

15. See, for example, Ginsburg and Rapp 1995; Foucault 1990; Blum 1993; Maher 1992; and Wolf 2010.

16. See Stacey (1983), Robinson (1985), Honig and Hershatter (1988), Rofel (2001), (2007), Croll (1981) and Wang (2003).

17. For discussions of changes in the way ideals of Chinese women have shifted and continue to change in the post-reform era, see Jin, Manning, and Chu 2006; and Wu 2010.

18. State-owned institutions generally provided health insurance, housing, subsidized foods, and services. Positions in them, in the 1990s, were still considered stable if low-paying jobs.

19. See appendix 1 for detailed background information on all the women in the study.

20. WHO Collaborative Study Team on the Role of Breastfeeding on the Prevention of Infant Mortality (2000). See also Morsy 1995 for an in-depth analysis of how such programs rationalize interventions into women's lives.

21. See Scheper-Hughes 1992 for a pioneering exception. In other areas of reproductive health, see works by Chapman (2003a, 2003b, 2010), Allen (2002), and Hausman (2010) for more recent contributions.

22. It was a great relief to find that others have struggled with this dilemma. Specifically, Kanaaneh (2002) in her study of reproduction among Palestinian women in Israel reinforced my decision to adopt this strategy and outlines in much more graceful terms the theoretical underpinnings of this dilemma.

23. See Parker and Dales 2015; Mahmood 2001; Jacka 2006; Ortner 2006; and Siti and Parker 2014 for discussions and case studies that demonstrate focusing on women's agency may not bring analytical clarity to our understanding of women's lives and in fact may obscure other ways of being and acting.

24. See Lock and Kaufert 1998. See Handwerker 1998 for insights into how Chinese women experiencing infertility navigate the imperative of having a child.

25. See the work of Lopez (2008), who shows that among Puerto Rican women in New York, women's decisions to undergo sterilization reflect multiple, coexisting, and temporal realities and histories. See also Cussins 1996; and Mol and Berg 1998.

26. See, for example, Ginsburg and Rapp 1995; Foucault 1979; Lupton 1995; Van Hollen 2003; Unnithan-Kumar 2004; Kanaaneh 2002; and Browner and Sargent 2011. This conceptualization builds on Anna Tsing's suggestion that anthropology can contribute to understanding globalization by documenting the changes in the social conditions and terrain that create possibilities for the circulation of people, ideas, objects, and institutions (2004, 463).

27. See Zhang and Ong 2008 for more recent cases describing the ways middle-class individuals fashion a sense of self within the constraints of China's capitalist economy. See Kuan 2015 for the dilemmas facing parents in twenty-first-century China as they encounter new demands of good parenthood in an increasingly competitive economic and social milieu.

28. See Zhu 2010 for insights into the negotiations between older and younger generations of women about nutrition during pregnancy.

29. See Hertz 1998 for an ethnographic perspective on the reopening of Shanghai's stock market.

30. Iron girls were role models in the Cultural Revolution who worked alongside men in the most physically demanding jobs—mining and construction, for example. These strong, capable women represented the efforts of the Chinese state under Mao Zedong to highlight women's equality in the workplace. See Jin, Manning, and Chu 2006.

31. Insurance provided to urban women covered the costs of prenatal care, hospital delivery, and postpartum care. The availability of this type of insurance has varied in the last twenty years.

32. See note 31.

33. See Schein 1999 for a full discussion of imagined cosmopolitanism in post-reform China.

34. See Evans 2010; Kuan 2015; Goodman 2014; Tomba 2009; and Duthie 2005.

35. For health care, see Duckett 2012; for urban China, see Davis et al. 1995.

36. For discussions and observations concerning the retreat of the state and civil society in the 1980s and early 1990s in China, see Solinger 1999; and Davis and Harrell 1993.

37. See also Greenhalgh 2008; and Greenhalgh and Winkler 2005.

38. See Greenhalgh and Winkler 2005; and Greenhalgh 2008 for analysis of the logic and rationale of the policy's implementation and iterations from the 1980s to the twenty-first century.

39. Peterson and Lupton (1997) document this trend in public health, also called the new public health. See also Chen 2001. However, as Greenhalgh shows, the one-child policy was always closely linked to China's economic modernization project (2010).

40. See, for example, Donath, Amir, and ALSPAC Study Team 2003; Lawson and Tulloch 1995; Lee et al. 2005; Mitra et al. 2004; and DiGirolamo et al. 2005.

Chapter One

1. On this incident, see International Baby Food Action Network. http://ibfan.org/fact-contaminants-reports-recall.

2. Thus, this study builds on research about the intersection between government intervention in reproduction in China and other parts of the world and the strategies used by ordinary people to order their lives in their own interests. See, for example, Andaya 2014; Greenhalgh 2008; Rivkin-Fish 2005; Murphy 2012; Browner and Sargent 2011; Van Hollen 2003, 2011; Allen 2004; Paxson 2004; and Kanaaneh 2002.

3. See also Apple 1987, 2006; and Golden 1996 for more historical analysis of infant feeding in the United States. See also Mink 1996 for more information about linking good mothers and breastfeeding to strengthening the nation as a world power.

4. See Mink 1996; Blum 1999; and Apple 2006.

5. See Apple 1987 for an extensive discussion about these developments.

6. Ibid.

7. Ibid.

8. See, for example, Trussell et al. 1992.

9. Ibid. See also Rudzik 2012 for a study that combines quantitative and ethnographic data about breastfeeding among low-income women in Brazil.

10. See Levine 1988 for a study documenting that rural Nepalese women involved in home-based work or agriculture used alternatives to breast milk.

11. Programs also exist in countries like the United States to promote breastfeeding among poor women. See Koerber 2013.

12. On a global level, low and declining rates of breastfeeding have been shown to be strongly associated with women's participation in paid employment (Wilmoth and Elder 1995; Popkin et al. 1986). Furthermore, those children most likely to succumb to malnutrition and disease have mothers with less schooling and unstable work situations. By contrast, women with more education and better jobs seem to be more likely to rear healthy children.

13. Notably, in the United States infant formula in 2005 was the fourth most commonly stolen good. It has a significant presence on the black market because it is a product for which there is constant demand (Clayton 2005).

14. See Wolf 2010. Most US states, European countries, and Canada provide mothers with subsidies for infant formula, although the criteria to obtain such assistance varies widely.

15. See ibid.; and Cassidy and El Tom 2014 for research on the properties of breast milk.

16. Disagreement exists about whether exclusive breastfeeding for four months is better than for six months. See Wolf 2010.

17. See Maher 1992; and Law 2000 for more sustained discussions.

18. A policy paper issued by China's State Council in 1996 outlines the situation of children and notes many advances in their well-being and health (Xinhua News Agency 1996b).

19. The United Nations Convention on the Elimination of All Forms of Discrimination against Women was ratified in China with some modifications. See McKenzie 1993. On a different level, China's push for admission to the WTO also stemmed from a pragmatic need to agree to conform to international standards.

20. China's bid to join and eventual entrance into the WTO is a well-known example of this.

21. Aside from China's Birth Planning Policy, the 1994 Maternal and Infant Health Law garnered a great deal of international attention within and outside China (see Dikotter 1998; and Greenhalgh and Winkler 2005) in part because the title of the draft law used the word *yousheng* 优生, which can be translated as "eugenics" but literally means "superior birth." The government later revised the name of the law to its current Maternal and Infant Health Law.

22. See Paxson 2004; Krause 2005; and Kanaaneh 2002.

23. See Rose 2007, 132.

24. See also Greenhalgh and Winkler 2005; and for a broader application Lupton 1995, 9.

25. Elise Andaya's work in Cuba (2014) shows how the state's interest in reducing infant mortality can come to be reflected in the practices of a local prenatal clinic.

26. At this time the policy was still strictly enforced. Greenhalgh and Winkler (2005) document the intensity and application of the policy across the regime changes since the its implementation. See Fong 2004 for an extended discussion of parental aspirations for their single children and Kuan 2015 for more recent dilemmas of parents in China.

27. See Molony 1995 for discussions on motherhood protection in Japan.

28. "Cat Theory: Contextualizing Deng Xiaoping's Pragmatisim," Shenzhen Noted: http://shenzhennoted.com/2012/08/22/cat-theory-contextualizing-deng-xiaopings-pragmatism/

29. For the text of the law, see http://www.china.org.cn/english/government/207405.htm

30. See Woo 1993 for an analysis of the law and its consequences for women.

31. See also Robinson 1985; and Short et al. 2002.

32. World Health Organization 1981. Observers and researchers since the late 1990s have noted that China's hospitals violate the law regularly.

33. Mead-Johnson sales representative, interview with the author, Beijing, 1995. The dominance of foreign companies continued in 2014, especially after the 2008 incident where formula contaminated with melamine caused widespread illness and a number of deaths. I wrote to the three formula companies with a prominent presence in the Beijing area but received no information regarding their sales or production.

34. See also Robinson 1985.
35. See also Notar 1994.

Chapter Two

1. See, for example, Otsuka et al. 2013; Hull, Thapa, and Wiknjosastro 1989; and Van Esterik 1989.

2. See Li et al. 2009; Rosenberg, Stull, and Adler 2008; Phillip and Merewood 2004; Baumslag and Michels 1995; Chetley 1986; Popkin et al. 1986.

3. Parts of this chapter are drawn from Gottschang 2000, 2001.

4. With the exception of the poster depicted in figure 2, the printed posters in the hallways of the Number 35 Hospital were mass-produced and contained primarily graphic (not photographic) images of women breastfeeding. Others were made by a talented relative of one of the nurses at the hospital. The poster in figure 2 advertises, at the bottom, a nutritional supplement based on Chinese traditional medicines for new mothers.

5. Maine lobsters were an imported rarity in China and if available cost more than one hundred US dollars in 1995.

6. All the women I observed during my fieldwork received nutritional pamphlets published by western formula companies.

7. Women received vitamin supplements as part of their prenatal care, but these were distributed by the hospital pharmacy with a prescription written by physicians.

8. See Zhu 2010 for an in-depth look at how pregnant women and their mothers negotiate and argue about nutrition during pregnancy in twenty-first-century China.

9. In recording the reactions to the film of all thirty women, these sequences represent those most frequently commented on in addition to material I chose to help contextualize them.

10. I watched the video with all the women in my study sample and, in addition to recording their spontaneous comments during the viewing, solicited their reactions after the presentation.

11. This logic draws on Andrew Strathern's argument that in biomedicine the biological is universal and culture is a limiting construct for individuals (1996, 145).

12. See Baumslag and Michels 1995.

13. See Chamberlain 1997.

14. See Gong and Jackson 2013; and Griffiths, Chapman, and Christiansen 2010.

15. See Dikotter 1998; Ferry 2001; and Greenhalgh ;2008.

16. See Gammeltoft 2014.

17. The "consumerist" body as an expression of self has been extensively

explored by Mike Featherstone (1991). See Ferry 2001; Dai 2002; and Ling 1999 on China, as well as Canclini 2001.

18. The connection between successful bodily management and social capital has been documented by scholars of China in a number of contexts. See Brownell 1995; Farquhar 2002; and Schein 1999. Matthew Kohrman illustrates the relationship between bodies and capital among disabled Chinese and shows that the long-standing traditional equation between bodily perfection and moral and spiritual status persists in China (2005, 120).

19. Uterine prolapse is a condition in which the middle portion of the uterus collapses and sometimes presses on the cervix. It can occur as a result of trauma experienced during childbirth.

20. See Chen 2001 for an account of this in 1990s Beijing.

21. In recent years scholars have begun to focus on the increasing income gap and its consequences for urban Chinese. See Zhang, Brym, and Anderson 2017.

22. *Peninsula City News,* November 2, 2011, quoted in Tang et al. 2014.

Chapter Three

1. See, for example, Andaya 2014; Ivry 2009; Davis-Floyd 2011; and Martin 1987.

2. In twenty-first-century urban China, women and their families have become much more invested in the medical care received during pregnancy. The rapid development of a number high-end private obstetrics hospitals, as well as private rooms and care in public hospitals, especially in China's coastal cities, attests to this change.

3. See Lutsiv et al. 2013b.

4. See Browner and Sargent 2011; Ivry 2009; Jasanoff 2004; and Jordan 1983.

5. See Sleeboom-Faulkner 2010; and Farquhar 2002 for discussions about popular medical books in China.

6. This phenomenon may be comparable to the Japanese concept of *amae,* which connotes a quality of dependence on others for one's well-being. Doi (1986) explains this concept of *amae* as one of central importance in mother-child interactions, which is most clearly illuminated in the mother's empathic understanding of a child's needs. More important, the relationship is not one-sided but becomes a reciprocal dynamic that can characterize relationships among adults as well (Vogel 1996).

7. See Zhu's (2010) research on intergenerational relations and pregnancy for an in-depth look at the negotiation of how best to maintain a healthy pregnancy. See also Andaya 2014; and Ivry 2009.

8. See also Honig and Hershatter 1988.

9. See Yan 2011 for more discussion of the increasing importance of the conjugal relationship in Chinese families.

10. Erbaugh (2000) notes that as modern Chinese families have become smaller, friendships among women (and men) have become increasingly important.

11. I met some women's husbands when I visited their homes or joined them for a social outing.

12. *Patrilineal* refers to a pattern of descent reckoned through males.

13. At some western-style private clinics in large cities, husbands are encouraged to participate in the labor and delivery process, and the practice of having a support person for the laboring woman is being studied and slowly introduced in some public hospitals. See Cheung et al. 2009.

14. The transmission of HIV from mother to fetus has provided insight into the conflict between maternal and fetal interests. See Kelly, Hampson, and Huff 2012.

15. "Little emperor" is a common phrase used to describe the spoiled single children that have grown up in China since the advent of the one-child policy.

16. See Zheng 2009; and Wallis 2013.

17. For Vietnam, see Zhu 2013; and Gammeltoft 2014.

18. See Greenhalgh 2008; and Zhu 2010.

Chapter Four

1. See, for example, Balogun et al. 2015 for a review and assessment of interventions to promote breastfeeding.

2. Apgar scores are used to determine the physical well-being of an infant and are performed at one and five minutes after birth. The criteria include skin color, heart rate, respiration, reflex responses, and muscle tone. Infants with low Apgar scores are likely to have neurological or respiratory problems (Consolini 1999).

3. See Gottschang 2016; Johnson and Wu 2015; Feng et al. 2011; Davis-Floyd 1992; Rothman 1991, and Sargent and Stark 1989.

4. Since the beginning of the twenty-first century, some hospitals in large cities have offered prenatal birthing support classes for couples and allowed the husband to be present at the birth. A more detailed account of childbirth at the Number 35 may be found in Gottschang, in preparation.

5. The average cost of a stay in a private room was six hundred yen or seventy-two US dollars.

6. See Chen 2012; Pillsbury 1978; Bao et al. 2010; Wang et al. 2008; and Callister 2006 for more studies on the ways women sit the month throughout the Chinese cultural sphere.

7. See Holroyd, Lopez, and Chan 2011 for more recent research on these practices.

8. Furth suggests that translating pollution into contagion may have "masked the cultural symbolism that made pollution ideas signposts of social and cosmic danger and tools for the restoration of order" (1987, 29). Furthermore, the medicalization of pollution suggests that the dangerous nature of disease may be controlled or mitigated through medical treatment, thus eliminating a social or symbolic threat (29).

9. See Yan 2011.

10. See Gottschang 2001, 2007, 2016; Robinson 1985; and Johnson 2011.

11. This narrative of avoiding sitting the month also appears in Gottschang 2016. As she was the only woman who did not sit the month, I rely on her narrative here as well.

12. See also Holroyd, Lopez, and Chan 2011; and Harvey and Buckley 2009.

13. See Lomoro et al. 2002 in which some Shanghai women register similar concerns.

14. I can discern few class differences in my study sample with regard to this phenomenon.

15. For more insights into women's bodies in 1990s China, see Evans 1997; Brownell 1995, Brownell and Wasserstrom 2002; and Gottschang 2001, 2007. Ip (2003) traces discussions about beauty and femininity in the Mao era and provides an important corrective to the idea that concern with feminine beauty is something that arrived in the post-Mao reform era.

16. Zhu (2010) examines the conflicts and mediation around food and pregnancy among middle-class Chinese women and their mothers.

17. Most women do not experience much leakage after the first few weeks of breastfeeding. During this research nursing pads, which protect women's clothing, were not readily available. In fact, I found them in only one Japanese-owned department store. By 1999, however, they were more easily found in large stores.

18. In their overview of childbirth in contemporary China, Harvey and Buckley explain the persistence of sitting the month in the twenty-first century as an instance of the older generation of mothers having "the authority to override the salient modernistic discourse and instead impose traditional customs to control the younger women's actions during this month" (2009, 64).

19. See also *China Daily* 2007.

20. In addition to these centers, a new set of sitting-the-month services has emerged in the context of China's twenty-first-century booming urban economy. These services include sitting-the-month nurses and attendants

who stay with new mothers in the home and food delivery services that provide alternatives or additions to the typical practices supervised by older female kin.

Chapter Five

1. See Andors 1983.

2. While these businesses were largely operated by individual women, family members often provided support by helping with deliveries, taking a shift, or helping with the work process.

3. These rates have fluctuated at times since 1949 when general unemployment was high. For example, in the early 1960s women were asked to give up their jobs so that men could find employment (Andors 1983). The rationale underlying this practice rested on the assumption that men were the family breadwinners and women could best serve the socialist cause by working as housewives. See also Honig and Hershatter 1988; and Solinger 1999.

4. One woman, Gu Lijian (see Chapter 3), did not want to breastfeed and did not try to do so.

5. See, for example, Popkin et al. 1986; and Merewood et al. 2005. For ethnographic approaches to breastfeeding that seek to complicate such studies, see Cassidy and El Tom 2014.

6. See Jelliffe and Jelliffe 1978 for this conclusion and Wolf 2010 for a summary of debates about this conclusion.

7. Traditionally, newborns were considered one year of age. Thus they were counted as 3 years old.

8. See also Masvie 2006; and Van Esterik 1995.

9. See Gussler and Briesemeister 1980; Greiner, Van Esterik, and Latham 1981; and Quandt 1995.

10. See Gatti 2008.

11. See Dettwyler and Macadam 1995; Van Esterik 1995, 2001; Rudzik 2012; and Scheper-Hughes 1992.

12. See the work of Teresa Kuan (2015), who studies the anxieties and practices of middle-class Chinese mothers as they rear their school-age children.

13. See also Strathern 1996, 21.

14. Infant formula was not actively or widely marketed in China during my research. However, stores in Beijing created rather dramatic displays by stacking cans of powdered or liquid formula in huge pyramids on their counters. Baby foods did not appear on Beijing's billboards, as I discovered during 1999, but subway stations throughout the city had Heinz baby food posters in prominent locations on the platforms.

15. At the time, 1996, Chinese families were hiring *bao mu* (children's

nurses) to care for their children, and indeed there was a specific street in Beijing where young women from the countryside would congregate and prospective employers could find someone to hire. Since then the practice has continued to grow, but agencies have sprung up to facilitate the hiring process.

16. Short et al. (2002) also find that among women wage laborers in China, child care is managed so as to accommodate work demands.

17. See also Evans 2010.

18. Research by scholars of China on issues of child development, child care, and parenting have become increasingly numerous in the last fifteen years, and I believe this reflects increasing popular concern with these issues. See, for example, Santos 2006.

19. See Fong 2004 for a detailed examination of expectations for China's only children.

20. See ibid.

21. See also Ma 2001.

22. See Robinson 1985; and Honig and Hershatter 1988.

23. See also Friedman 2006.

Conclusion

1. See Rivkin-Fish's (2005) study of this process in Russia and Gammeltoft's (2014) in Vietnam.

2. The efficacy of policies and regulations designed to assist mothers in the workplace is still contested. See McLeod, Pullson, and Cookson 2002; and Cooklin, Donath, and Amir 2008, 623.

References

Abrahams, S., and M. Labbok. 2009. "Exploring the Impact of the Baby-Friendly Hospital Initiative on Trends in Exclusive Breastfeeding." *International Breastfeeding Journal* 4:11.

Ahern, Emily. 1975. "The Power and Pollution of Chinese Women." In *Women in Chinese Society,* edited by Marjory Wolf and Roxanne Witke, 193–214. Palo Alto, CA: Stanford University Press.

Allen, Denise Roth. 2004 *Managing Motherhood, Managing Risk: Fertility and Danger in West Central Tanzania.* Ann Arbor: University of Michigan Press.

Amir, Lisa H. 2011. "Breastfeeding and Social Theory." *International Breastfeeding Journal* 6:7.

Anagnost, Ann. 1995. "A Surfeit of Bodies: Population and the Rationality of the State in Post-Mao China." In *Conceiving the New World Order: The Global Politics of Reproduction,* edited by Faye Ginsburg and Rayna Rapp, 22–41. Berkeley: University of California Press.

Andaya, Elise. 2014. *Conceiving Cuba: Reproduction, Women, and the State in the Post-Soviet Era.* New Brunswick, NJ: Rutgers University Press.

Andors, Phyllis. 1983. *The Unfinished Liberation of Chinese Women.* Bloomington: Indiana University Press.

Apple, Rima. 1987. *Mothers and Medicine: A Social History of Infant Feeding, 1890–1950.* Madison: University of Wisconsin Press.

Apple, Rima. 2006. *Perfect Motherhood: Science and Childbearing in America.* New Brunswick NJ: Rutgers University Press.

Armstrong, David. 1995. "The Rise of Surveillance Medicine." *Sociology of Health and Illness* 17(3): 393–404.

Armstrong, Elizabeth. 2002. "Lessons in Control: Prenatal Education in the Hospital." *Social Problems* 47(4): 583–605.

Aubel, J. 2012. "The Role and Influence of Grandmothers on Child Nutrition: Culturally Designated Advisors and Caregivers." *Maternal and Child Nutrition* 8:19–35.

Awofeso, N. 2004. "What's New about the 'New' Public Health?" *American Journal of Public Health* 94(5): 705–9.

Balogun, O. O., A. Dagvadorj, K. M. Anigo, E. Ota, and S. Sasaki. 2015. "Factors Influencing Breastfeeding Exclusivity during the First Six Months of Life in Developing Countries: A Quantitative and Qualitative Systematic Review." *Maternal and Child Nutrition* 11(4): 433–51.

Bao, W., A. Ma, L. Mao, J. Lai, M. Xiao, G. Sun, Y. Ouyang, S. Wu, W. Yang, N. Wang, Y. Zhao, J. Fu, and L. Liu. 2010. "Diet and Lifestyle Interventions in Postpartum Women in China: Study Design and Rationale of a Multicenter Randomized Controlled Trial." *BMC Health* 103"1-8, doi: 10.1186/1471–2458–10–103.

Bauer, John, Wang Feng, Nancy Riley, and Xiaohua Zhao. 1992. "Gender Inequality in Urban China: Education and Employment." *Modern China* 18(3): 330–70.

Baumslag, Naomi, and Dia Michels. 1995. *Milk, Money, and Madness: The Culture and Politics of Breastfeeding.* Westport: CT: Bergin and Garvey.

Beijing Review. 2001. "Women's Choice: Home or Work?" April 25, 2001. http://www.china.org.cn/english/2001/Apr/11788.htm

Berkow, Robert, ed. 1982. *The Merck Manual.* 14th ed. Rahway, NJ: Merck Sharp and Dohme Research Laboratories.

Blum, Linda. 1993. "Mothers, Babies, and Breastfeeding in Late Capitalist America: The Shifting Contexts of Feminist Theory." *Feminist Studies* 19(2): 291–311.

Blum, Linda. 1999. *At the Breast: Ideologies of Breastfeeding and Motherhood in the Contemporary United States.* Boston: Beacon.

Bordo, Susan. 1993. *Unbearable Weight: Feminism, Western Culture, and the Body.* Berkeley: University of California Press.

Bourdieu, Pierre. 1977. *Outline of a Theory of Practice.* Cambridge: Cambridge University Press.

Bourdieu, Pierre. 1986. *Distinction.* Cambridge: Cambridge University Press.

Brahmbhatt, Heena, and Ronald Gray. 2000. "The Role of Breastfeeding in Preventing Infant Mortality." *Lancet* 355(9212): 1370.

Bray, Francesca. 1997. *Technology and Gender: Fabrics of Power in Late Imperial China.* Berkeley: University of California Press.

Brownell, Susan. 1995. *Training the Body for China: Sports in the Moral Order of the People's Republic.* Chicago: University of Chicago Press.

Brownell, Susan, and Jeffrey Wasserstrom. 2002. "Introduction: Theorizing Masculinities and Femininities." In *Chinese Femininities and Masculinities,* edited by Susan Brownell and Jeffrey Wasserstrom, 1–42. Berkeley: University of California Press.

Browner, Carole H., and Carolyn F. Sargent, eds. 2011. *Reproduction, Globalization, and the State: New Theoretical and Ethnographic Perspectives.* Durham, NC: Duke University Press.

Cai, Wenwei, James S. Marks, Charles H. C. Chen, Youxian Zhuang, Leo Morris, and Jeffrey Harris. 1998. "Increased Cesarean Section Rates and Emerging Patterns of Health Insurance in Shanghai, China. *American Journal of Public Health* 88(5): 777–80.

Callister, L. C. 2006. "Doing the Month: Chinese Postpartum Practices." *American Journal of Maternal and Child Nursing* 31(6): 390.

Canclini, Néstor Garcıá. 2001. *Consumers and Citizens: Globalization and Multicultural Conflicts.* Translated by George Yúdice. Minneapolis: University of Minnesota Press.

Carter, Pam. 1995. *Feminism, Breasts, and Breastfeeding.* New York: Palgrave Macmillan.

Cassidy Tanya, and Abdullahi El Tom, eds. 2014. *Ethnographies of Breastfeeding: Cultural Contexts and Confrontations.* London: Bloomsbury.

Catteneo, A. 2012. "Inequalities and Inequities in Breastfeeding: An International Perspective." *Breastfeeding Medicine* 7(1): 3–9. Academy of Breastfeeding Medicine Founder's Lecture, 2011.

Chamberlain, M. 1997. "A Baby-Friendly Hospital Initiative in Northern China." *Nursing Ethics* 4(6): 511–18.

Champagne, Susan. 1992. "Producing the Intelligent Child: Intelligence and the Child Rearing Discourse in the People's Republic of China." PhD diss., Stanford University.

Chapman, Rachel R. 2003a. "*A Nova Vida:* The Commoditization of Reproductive Health in Central Mozambique." *Medical Anthropology* 23(3): 229–61.

Chapman, Rachel R. 2003b. "Endangering Safe Motherhood in Mozambique: Prenatal Care as Pregnancy Risk. *Social Science and Medicine* 57(2): 355–74.

Chapman, Rachel R. 2010. *Family Secrets: Risking Reproduction in Central Mozambique.* Nashville, TN: Vanderbilt University Press.

Chen, Nancy. 2001. "Health, Wealth, and the Good Life in Urban China." In *China Urban: Ethnographies of Contemporary Culture,* edited by Nancy Chen, Constance Clark, Suzanne Gottschang, and Lyn Jeffrey, 165–82. Durham, NC: Duke University Press.

Chen, Sanna. 2012. *Zuo Yue Zi Sitting the Month in Taiwan: Implications for Intergenerational Relations.* Ann Arbor: Dissertation Abstracts International, University of Michigan.

Chen Ya. 1996. "Breastfeeding Promotion in China." *Beijing Review,* August 25, 15–16.

Chen, Yue. 1992. "Factors Associated with Artificial Feeding in Shanghai." *American Journal of Public Health* 82(2): 264–66.

Chetley, Andrew. 1986. *The Politics of Baby Foods: Successful Challenges to an International Marketing Strategy*. London: F. Pinter.

Cheung, Anthony B. L. 2001. "Health Policy Reform." In *The Market in Chinese Social Policy*, edited by Linda Wong and Norman Flynn, 63–87. New York: Palgrave.

Cheung, Ngai Fen, Rosemary Mander, Xiaoli Wang, Wei Fu, and Junghong Zhu. 2009. "Chinese Midwives' Views on a Proposed Midwife-Led Normal Birth Unit." *Midwifery* 25:744–55.

China Daily. 2007. "Health Center Gears Up to Pamper New Moms." February 14. http://english1.china.org.cn/english/health/200081.htm

China Daily, Xinhua News Agency. 2015. "Death of New Mother Stirs Doubts of Age-Old Practice." August 7. http://www.chinadaily.com.cn/china/2015-08/07/content_21532349.htm

China Statistical Bureau. 1994. *Statistical Yearbook of China*. Beijing: China Statistics Press.

Chinese Health Statistics Digest. 1995. In Therese Hesketh and Wei Xingzhu. 1997. "Maternal and Child Health in China."*British Medical Journal* 314(7098): 1898–1901.

Clayton, Mark. 2005. "Is Black Market Infant Formula Financing Terror?" *Christian Science Monitor*, June 29. Accessed March 21, 2013. http://www.csmonitor.com/2005/0629/p01s01-usju.html

Cohen, Anthony. 1994. *Self-Consciousness: An Alternative Anthropology of Identity*. New York: Routledge.

Consolini, Deborah. 1999. "Initial Care of the Newborn." In *Merck Manual of Diagnosis and Therapy* (online), edited by Mark Beers and Robert Berkow. Whitehouse Station, NJ: Merck.

Cooklin, Amanda R., Susan Donath, and Lisa Amir. 2008. "Maternal Employment and Breastfeeding: Results from the Longitudinal Study of Australian Children." *Acta Paediatrica* 97:620–23.

Croll, Elizabeth. 1981. *The Politics of Marriage in Contemporary China*. Cambridge: Cambridge University Press.

Cussins, Charis. 1996. "Ontological Choreography: Agency through Objectification in Infertility Clinics." *Social Studies of Science* 26:575–610.

Dai, Jinhua. 2002. "National Identity in the Hall of Mirrors." In *Cinema and Desire: Feminist Marxism and Cultural Politics in the Works of Dai Jinhua*, edited by Jing Wang and Tani E. Barlow, 189–212. London: Verso.

Dankert, G., H. Page, I. Qian, and R. Yang. 1991. Infant Feeding Practices in Hebei, Shaanxi, and Shanghai: Is Breastfeeding Declining or Is It Increasing? *Journal of Family Planning* 21(3): 78–91.

Davies-Adetugbo, A. A. 1997. "Sociocultural Factors and the Promotion of Exclusive Breastfeeding in Rural Yoruba Communities of Osun State, Nigeria." *Social Science and Medicine* 45:113–25.

Davis Deborah. 2000. *The Consumer Revolution in Urban China.* Berkeley: University of California Press.

Davis, Deborah, and Stevan Harrell, eds. 1993. *Chinese Families in the Post Mao Era.* Berkeley: University of California Press.

Davis, Deborah, Richard Kraus, Barry Naughton, and Elizabeth J. Perry, eds. 1995. *Urban Spaces in Contemporary China: The Potential for Autonomy and Community in Post-Mao China.* Cambridge: Cambridge University Press.

Davis-Floyd, Robbie. 1992. *Birth as an American Rite of Passage.* Berkeley: University of California Press.

Davis-Floyd, Robbie. 2011. "Birthing a Mother: The Surrogate Body and the Pregnant Self." *Birth* 38:180–81.

de Certeau, Michel. 1984. *The Practice of Everyday Life.* Berkeley: University of California Press.

Declercq E., Labbok M., Sakala C. 2009. "Hospital Practices and Women's Likelihood of Fulfilling their Intention to Exclusively Breastfeed." *American Journal of Public Health* 99:929–35.

Dettwyler Katherine A. 1987. "Breastfeeding and Weaning in Mali: Cultural Context and Hard Data." *Social Science and Medicine* 24(8): 633–44.

Dettwyler, Katherine, and Claudia Fishman. 1992. "Infant Feeding Practices and Growth." *Annual Review of Anthropology* 21:171–200.

DiGirolamo, A., N. Thompson, R. Martorelli, S. Fein, and L. Grummer-Strawn. 2005. "Intention or Experience? Predictors of Continued Breastfeeding." *Health Education and Behavior* 32:208–26.

Dikotter, Frank. 1995. *Sex, Culture, and Modernity in China: Medical Science and the Construction of Sexual Identities in the Early Republican Period.* London: Hurst.

Dikotter, Frank. 1998. *Imperfect Conceptions: Medical Knowledge, Birth Defects, and Eugenics in China.* New York: Columbia University Press.

Doi, L. Takeo. 1986. "Amae: A Key Concept for Understanding Japanese Personality Structure." In *Japanese Culture and Behavior: Selected Readings,* edited by Takie Lebra and William P. Libra. Honolulu: University of Hawai'i Press.

Donath, S. M., L. H. Amir, and the ALSPAC Study Team. 2003. "Relationship between Prenatal Feeding Intention and Duration of Breastfeeding: A Cohort Study." *Acta Paediatrica* 92:352–56.

Douglas, Mary. 1986. *Purity and Danger: An Analysis of Concepts of Pollution and Taboo.* Boston: Ark Paperbacks.

Du, Ren. 1992. *Ren Shen Yu Fen Mian Da Quan* 妊娠于分娩大全 [The complete book of pregnancy and birth]. Beijing: China Education Press.

Duckett, Jane. 2012. *The Chinese State's Retreat from Health.* New York: Routledge.

Duthie, Laurie. 2005. "White Collars with Chinese Characteristics: Global Capitalism and the Formation of Social Identities." *Anthropology of Work Review* 26(3): 1–11.

Dykes, Fiona, and Victoria Hall Moran. 2009 *Infant and Young Child Feeding: Challenges to Implementing a Global Strategy*. New York: Wiley.

Erbaugh, Mary S. 2000. "Greeting Cards in China: Mixed Language of Connections and Affections." In *The Consumer Revolution in Urban China,* edited by Deborah Davis, 171–200. Berkeley: University of California Press.

Erwin, Kathleen. 2000. "Heart-to-Heart, Phone-to-Phone: Family Values, Sexuality, and the Politics of Shanghai's Advice Hotlines." In *The Consumer Revolution in Urban China,* edited by Deborah Davis, 145–70. Berkeley: University of California Press.

Eurofood. 1996. "Potential for Growth in Chinese Baby Food Sector." *Eurofood,* May 22, 3.

Evans, Harriet. 1994. "Defining Difference: The Scientific Construction of Gender and Sexuality in the People's Republic of China." *Signs: Journal of Women, Culture, and Society* 20(2): 357–406.

Evans, Harriet. 1997. *Women and Sexuality in China.* New York: Continuum.

Evans, Harriet. 2010. "The Gender of Communication: Changing Expectations of Mothers and Daughters." *China Quarterly* 204:980–1000.

Evans, Harriet. 2011. *Gender in Flux: Agency and Its Limits in Contemporary China.* Cambridge: Cambridge University Press.

Fan Yiying. 2015. "Sitting the Month: Gift or Torture?" *What's on Weibo.* May 11. http://www.whatsonweibo.com/sitting-the-month/

Farquhar, Judith. 1987. "Problems of Knowledge in Contemporary Chinese Medical Discourse." *Social Science and Medicine* 24(12): 1013–21.

Farquhar, Judith. 2002. *Appetites: Food and Sex in Post-socialist China.* Durham, NC: Duke University Press.

Farquhar, Judith, and Qicheng Zhang. 2005. "Bio-political Beijing: Pleasure, Sovereignty, and Self-Cultivation in China's Capital." *Cultural Anthropology* 20(3): 303–27.

Featherstone, Mike. 1991. *Consumer Culture and Postmodernism.* London: Sage.

Feng X.L., S. Guo, D. Hipgrave, J. Zhu, L. Zhang, L. Song, Q. Yang, Y. Guo, and C. Ronsmans. 2011. "China's Facility-Based Birth Strategy and Neonatal Mortality: A Population-Based Epidemiological Study." *Lancet,* 378(9801): 1493–1500. doi:10.1016/S0140-6736(11)61096-9. Epub 2011 Sep 15.

Ferry, Megan. 2001. "Advertising, Consumerism, and Nostalgia for the New Woman in Contemporary China." *Continuum: Journal of Media and Cultural Studies* 17(3): 277–90.

Fong, Vanessa . 2004. *Only Hope: Coming of Age under China's One-Child Policy.* Palo Alto, CA: Stanford University Press.

Foucault, Michel. 1979. *Discipline and Punish: The Birth of the Prison.* New York: Vintage Books.Foucault, Michel. 1986. "Technologies of the Self." In *Technologies of the Self: A Seminar with Michel Foucault,* edited by Luther Martin, Huck Gutman, and Patrick Hutton, 16–49. Amherst: University of Massachusetts Press.

Foucault, Michel. 1990. *The History of Sexuality: An Introduction.* New York: Vintage.

Foucault, Michel. 2007. *Lectures at the College de France Security, Territory, Population.* New York: Palgrave McMillan.

Fouts, Hilary, Barry Hewlitt, and Michael Lamb. 2012. "A Biocultural Approach to Infant Feeding in Central Africa." *American Anthropologist* 114(1): 123–26.

Franklin, Sarah, Celia Lury, and Jackie Stacey, eds. 2000. *Global Nature, Global Culture.* Thousand Oaks, CA: Sage.

Fraser, David. 2000. "Inventing Oasis: Luxury Housing Advertisements and Reconfiguring Domestic Space in Shanghai." In *The Consumer Revolution in China,* edited by Deborah Davis, 25–53. Berkeley: University of California Press.

Friedman, Sara. 2006. *Intimate Politics: Marriage, the Market, and State Power in Southeastern China.* Cambridge, MA: Harvard University Press.

Furth, Charlotte. 1987. "Concepts of Pregnancy, Childbirth, and Infancy in Ch'ing Dynasty China." *Journal of Asian Studies* 46:7–36.

Furth, Charlotte. 1999. *A Flourishing Yin: Gender in China's Medical History, 960–1665.* Berkeley: University of California Press.

Gammeltoft, Tine M. 2013. "Potentiality and Human Temporality: Haunting Futures in Vietnamese Pregnancy Care." *Current Anthropology* 54(suppl. 7): S159–71.

Gammeltoft, Tine M. 2014. *Haunting Images: A Cultural Account of Selective Reproduction in Vietnam.* Berkeley: University of California Press.

Gan, Li. 2013. "Findings from China Household Finance Survey." Texas A&M University and Southwestern University of Finance and Economics, China Household Finance Survey Working paper. http://people.tamu.edu/~ganli/Report-English-Dec-2013.pdf

Gastaldo, Denise. 1997. "Is Health Education Good for You? Re-thinking Health Education through the Concept of Bio-Power." In *Foucault, Health, and Medicine,* edited by Alan Petersen and Robin Bunton, 114–33. New York: Routledge.

Gates, Hill. 1995. "Cultural Support for Birth Limitation among Urban, Capital-Owning Women." In *Chinese Families in the Post-Mao Era,* edited by Deborah Davis and Stevan Harrell, 251–76. Berkeley: University of California Press.

Gatti, Lisa J. 2008. "Maternal Perceptions of Insufficient Milk Supply in Breastfeeding." *Journal of Nursing Scholarship* 40(4): 355–63.

Geddes, Donna T. 2007. "Inside the Lactating Breast: The Latest Research." *Journal of Midwifery and Women's Health* 52(6): 556–63.

Giddens, Anthony. 1979. *Central Problems in Social Theory: Action, Structure, and Contradiction in Social Analysis.* London: Macmillan.

Giddens, Anthony. 1991. *Modernity and Self-identity: Self and Society in the Late Modern Age.* Stanford, CA: Stanford University Press.

Ginsburg, Faye, and Rayna Rapp. 1991. "The Politics of Reproduction." *Annual Review of Anthropology* 20:311–43.

Ginsburg, Faye, and Rayna Rapp, eds. 1995. "Introduction." In *Conceiving the New World Order: The Global Politics of Reproduction,* 1–19. Berkeley: University of California Press.

Glosser, Susan. 1999. "Milk for Health, Milk for Profit: Shanghai's Chinese Dairy Industry under Japanese Occupation." In *Inventing Nanjing Road: Commercial Culture in Shanghai, 1900–1945,* edited by Sherman Cochran, 207–33. Ithaca, NY: East Asia Program, Cornell University.

Golden, Janet. 1996. *A Social History of Wet Nursing in America: From Breast to Bottle.* Cambridge: Cambridge University Press.

Gong, Qian, and Peter Jackson. 2013. "Mediating Science and Nature: Representing and Consuming Infant Formula Advertising in China." *European Journal of Cultural Studies* 16(3): 285–309.

Goodman, David. 2014. *Class in Contemporary China.* Cambridge, UK: Polity.

Gordon, Deborah. 1988. "Tenacious Assumptions in Western Medicine." In *Biomedicine Examined,* edited by Margaret Lock and Deborah Gordon, 19–56. Dordrecht: Kluwer.

Gottschang, Suzanne. 2000. "A Baby Friendly Hospital and the Science of Infant Feeding." In *Feeding China's Little Emperors: Food, Culture, and Social Change,* edited by Jing Jun, 160–84. Palo Alto, CA: Stanford University Press.

Gottschang, Suzanne. 2001. "The Consuming Mother: Infant Feeding and the Feminine Body in Urban China." In *China Urban: Ethnographies of Contemporary Culture,* edited by Nancy Chen, Constance Clark, Suzanne Gottschang, and Lyn Jeffrey, 89–103. Durham, NC: Duke University Press.

Gottschang, Suzanne. 2007. "Maternal Bodies, Breastfeeding and Consumer Desire in Urban China." *Medical Anthropology Quarterly* 21(1): 64–80.

Gottschang, Suzanne. 2016. "Taking Patriarchy out of Postpartum Recovery?" In *Transformations of Chinese Patriarchy,* edited by Stevan Harrell and Goncalo Santos, 201–18. Seattle: University of Washington Press.

Gottschang, Suzanne. 2017. "Spaces of Care: Childbirth in a Chinese Hospital." In preparation.

Greenhalgh, Susan. 1990. "Evolution of the One-Child Policy in Shaanxi, 1979–1988." *China Quarterly* 122:191–34.

Greenhalgh, Susan. 1993. "Controlling Births and Bodies in Village China." *American Ethnologist* 21(1): 233–56.

Greenhalgh, Susan. 2003. "Planned Births, Unplanned Persons: "Population" in the Making of Chinese Modernity." *American Ethnologist* 30(2): 196–215.

Greenhalgh, Susan. 2005. "Globalization and Population Governance in China." In *Global Assemblages: Technology, Politics, and Ethics as Anthropological Problems,* edited by Aihwa Ong and Stephen J. Collier, 354–72. Malden, MA: Blackwell.

Greenhalgh, Susan. 2008. *Just One Child: Science and Policy in Deng's China.* Berkeley: University of California Press.

Greenhalgh, Susan. 2010. *Cultivating Global Citizens: Population in the Rise of China.* Edwin O. Reischauer Lecture, 2008. Cambridge, MA: Harvard University Press.

Greenhalgh, Susan, and Edward Winkler. 2005. *Governing China's Population: From Leninist to Neoliberal Biopolitics.* Berkeley: University of California Press.

Greiner, Ted, Penny Van Esterik, and Michael Latham. 1981. "Commentary: The Insufficient Milk Syndrome; an Alternative Explanation. *Medical Anthropology* 5(2): 233–47.

Griffiths, Michael B., Malcolm Chapman, and Flemming Christiansen. 2010. "Chinese Consumers: The Romantic Reappraisal." *Ethnography* 11(3): 331–57.

Gussler, Judith, and Linda Briesemeister. 1980. "The Insufficient Milk Syndrome: A Biocultural Explanation." *Medical Anthropology* 4(2): 145–74.

Guo, Sufang, Xulan Fu, Robert W. Scherpbier, Yan Wang, Hong Zhou, Xiaoli Wang, and David B. Hipgrave. 2013. "Breastfeeding Rates in Central and Western China in 2010: Implications for Child and Population Health." *Bulletin of the World Health Organization* 91:322–31.

Halvorson, G. C. 1992. *Strong Medicine.* New York: Random House.

Handwerker, Lisa. 1998. "The Consequences of Modernity for Childless Women in China: Medicalization and Resistance." In *Pragmatic Women and Body Politics,* edited by Margaret Lock and Patricia A. Kaufert, 178–205. Cambridge: Cambridge University Press.

Hanser, Amy, and Jialin Camille Li. 2015. "Opting Out? Gated Consumption, Infant Formula, and China's Affluent Urban Consumers." *China Journal* 74:110–28.

Harney, Rebecca. 2013. "Special Report: How Big Formula Bought China." Reuters News Agency, November 8. http://www.reuters.com/article/2013/11/08/us-china-milkpowder-specialreport-idUSBRE9A700820131108

Harvey, Travis, and Lila Buckley. 2009. "Childbirth in China." In *Childbirth across Cultures,* edited by Helaine Selin and Pamela Stone, 55–70. New York: Springer.

Hausman, Bernice. 2010. *Viral Mothers: Breastfeeding in the Age of HIV/AIDS.* Ann Arbor: University of Michigan Press.

Henderson, Gail, and Barbara Entwistle. 1994. "Gender and Family Business in Rural China." *American Sociological Review* 60(1): 36–58.

Hertz, Ellen. 1998. *The Trading Crowd: An Ethnography of the Shanghai Stock Market.* Cambridge: Cambridge University Press.

Higgs, Paul. 1994. "Risk, Governmentality, and the Reconceptualization of Citizenship." In *Modernity, Medicine, and Health,* edited by Graham Scambler and Paul Higgs, 177–98. New York: Routledge.

Hird, M. J. 2007. "The Corporeal Generosity of Maternity." *Body and Society* 13(1): 1–20.

Holroyd, Eleanor, Violetta Lopez, and Sally Wai-Chi Chan. 2011. "Negotiating 'Doing the Month': An Ethnographic Study Examining Postnatal Practices of Two Generations of Chinese Women." *Nursing Health Science* 13(1): 47–52.

Hong Qin, Lin Zhang, Lingling Zhang, Wei Zhang, Li Li, Xin Deng, Danping Tian, Jing Deng, and Guoqing Hu. 2017. "Prevalence of Breastfeeding: Findings from the First Health Service Household Interviewing, Hunan Province, China." *International Journal of Environmental Research and Public Health* 14(150): 1–8, doi:10.3390/ijerph14020150.

Honig, Emily, and Gail Hershatter. 1988. *Personal Voices: Chinese Women in the 1980's.* Stanford, CA: Stanford University Press.

Huffman, Sandra L. 1984. "Determinants of Breastfeeding in Developing Countries: Overview and Policy Implications." *Studies in Family Planning* 15(4): 170–83.

Hull, Valerie, Shyam Thapa, and Gulardi Wiknjosastro. 1989. "Breastfeeding and Health Professionals: A Study in Hospitals in Indonesia." *Social Science and Medicine* 20(4): 355–64.

Ingram, J., D. Johnson, and N. Hamid. 2003. "South Asian Grandmothers' Influence on Breastfeeding in Bristol." *Midwifery* 12(2003): 318–27.

Ip Hung-Yok. 2003. "Fashioning Appearances: Feminine Beauty in Chinese Communist Revolutionary Culture. *Modern China* 29(3): 329–61.

Ivry, Tsipy. 2009. *Embodying Culture: Pregnancy in Japan and Israel.* New Brunswick, NJ: Rutgers University Press.

Jacka, Tamara. 1990. "Back to the Wok: Women and Employment in Chinese Industry in the 1980s." *Australian Journal of Chinese Affairs* 24:1–23.

Jacka, Tamara. 1997. *Women's Work in Rural China: Change and Continuity in an Era of Reform.* Cambridge: Cambridge University Press.

Jacka, Tamara. 2006. *Rural Women in Urban China: Gender, Migration, and Social Change.* Armonk, NY: M. E. Sharpe.

Jagger, Allison. 1983. *Feminist Politics and Human Nature.* New York: Rowman and Littlefield.

Jasanoff, Sheila. 2004. "The Idiom of Co-Production." In *States of Knowledge in the Co-production of Science and the Social Order,* edited by Sheila Jasanoff, 1–12. New York: Routledge.

Jelliffe, D. B., and E. F. P. Jelliffe. 1978. *Human Milk in the Modern World.* Oxford: Oxford University Press.

Jin Yihong, Kimberly Manning, and Lianyun Chu. 2006. "Rethinking the 'Iron Girls': Gender and Labour during the Chinese Cultural Revolution." *Gender and History* 18:613–34.

Johnson, Tina. 2011. *Childbirth in Republican China: Delivering Modernity.* Lanham, MD: Lexington.

Jordon, Brigitte. 1983. *Birth in Four Cultures.* Montreal: Eden.

Kanaaneh, Rhoda. 2002. *Birthing the Nation: Strategies of Palestinian Women in Israel.* Berkeley: University of California Press.

Kelly, Kristin, Sarah C. Hampson, and Jamie Huff. 2012. "Prenatal HIV Testing: The Compartmentalization of Women's Sexual Risk Exposure and the Return of the Maternal Fetal Conflict." *Women and Health* 52(7): 700–715.

Kim Won, S., V. Fong, H. Yoshikawa, N. Way, X. Chen, H. Deng, and Z. Lu. 2010. "Income, Work Preferences, and Gender Roles among Parents of Infants in Urban China: A Mixed Method Study from Nanjing." *China Quarterly* 204:939–59, doi:10.1017/S0305741010001037.

Kipnis, Andrew. 2012. *Chinese Modernity and the Individual Psyche.* New York: Palgrave MacMillan.

Kleinman, Arthur, Yunxiang Yan, Jing Jun, Sing Lee, and Everett Zhang. 2011. *Deep China: The Moral Life of the Person.* Berkeley: University of California Press.

Koerber, Amy. 2103. *Breast or Bottle? Contemporary Controversies in Infant Feeding Policy and Practice.* Columbia: University of South Carolina Press.

Kohrman, Matthew. 2005. *Bodies of Difference: Experiences of Disability and Institutional Advocacy in the Making of Modern China.* Berkeley: University of California Press.

Krause, Betsey. 2005. *A Crisis of Births: Population Politics and Family-Making in Italy.* Case Studies on Contemporary Social Issues. Belmont, CA: Wadsworth.

Kristof, Nicholas. 2015. "The Breast Milk Elixir." *New York Times,* October 22. https://www.nytimes.com/2015/10/22/opinion/the-miracle-breast-milk-elixir.html

Kuan, Teresa. 2015. *Love's Uncertainty: The Politics and Ethics of Childrearing in Contemporary China.* Berkeley: University of California Press.

Kwan, Coldness. 2006. "High-Paid Professional Wet Nurse Stirs Debate." *China Daily* June 30. http://www.chinadaily.com.cn/china/2006-06/30/content_630610.htm

Law, Jules. 2000. "The Politics of Breastfeeding: Assessing Risk and Dividing Labor." *Signs: Journal of Women in Culture and Society* 25(2): 407–50.

Lawson, K., and M. I. Tulloch. 1995. "Breastfeeding Duration: Prenatal Intentions and Postnatal Practices." *Journal of Advanced Nursing* 22:841–49.

Layne, Linda. 1999. *Transformative Motherhood.* New York: New York University Press.

Lee, H., M. Rubio, I. Elo, K. McCollum, E. Chung, and J. Culhane. 2005. "Factors Associated with Intention to Breastfeed among Low-Income, Inner-City Pregnant Women. *Maternal and Child Health Journal* 9:253–61.

Lei, Xiong. 1997. "China Media: TV Ads Depict Women as Helpless and Weak." *Interpress Service,* April 29.

Levin, Dan. 2015. A Tradition for New Mothers Now $27,000 a Month. *New York Times,* October 1. https://www.nytimes.com/2015/10/02/business/international/china-confinement-care-for-new-mothers-now-27000-a-month.html?_r=0

Levine, Nancy. 1988. "Women's Work and Infant Feeding: A Case from Nepal." *Ethnology* 27(3): 231–51.

Li, An Le, and Li Hong An, eds. 1991. *Huai yun qian hou hua you sheng* 怀孕前后话优胜 [Before and after pregnancy: Observations on good nurturing]. Beijing: Zhongguo Renkou Chubenshe.

Li, Victor H. 1975. "Politics and Health Care in China: The Barefoot Doctors." *Stanford Law Review* 27(3): 827–40.

Li, X.-Y., H.-L. Zhang, and S.-Q. Dong. 2005. "Influence Factor Study of Quality of Life for Postpartum Women." *Chinese Health Service Management* 21(4): 235–37.

Li Zhen, Bai Shuguang, Wang Wenyue, and Hou ShuFeng. 2009. "Changchun City Maternal and Child Health Care Worker's Knowledge of Infant Feeding: An Assessment of the Current Situation and Future Directions." *Maternal and Child Health Care of China* 7:20–24.

Liamputtong, Pranee. 2007. "Childrearing and Infant Care Issues: A Cross Cultural Perspective." In *Childrearing and Infant Care Issues: A Cross Cultural Perspective,* edited by Pranee Liamputtong, 3–29. New York: Nova Science Publishers.

Ling, L. H. M. 1999. "Sex Machine: Global Hypermasculinity and Images of the Asian Woman in Modernity." *positions: east asia cultures critique* 7(2): 277–306.

Liu, A., Y. Dai, X. Xie, and L. Chen. 2014. "Implementation of International Code of Marketing Breast-Milk Substitutes in China." *Breastfeeding Medicine* 9(9): 467–72.

Liu, Jianghong, Ai-Ling Ji, Yinling Irene Wong, and Tongjian Cai. 2014. "Infant formula Safety Concerns and Consequences in China." *World Journal of Pediatrics* 10(1): 7–9.

Liu, Jieyu. 2007. *Gender and Work in Urban China: Women Workers of the Unlucky Generation.* London: Routledge.

Liu, Wei. 2016. "Baby-Friendly Hospital Initiative and Reassessment." Paper presented at the at Baby-Friendly Hospital Initiative Congress, WHO, Geneva, Switzerland, October 24.

Liu, Yanqun, Maria Petrini, and Judith Maloni. 2015. "Doing the Month: Post-partum Practices in Chinese Women." *Nursing and Health Services* 17:5–14.

Lock, Jean. 1986. "Effect of Ideology in Gender Role Definition: China as a Case Study." *Journal of Asian and African Studies* 24(3–4): 228–38.

Lock, Margaret, and Patricia Kaufert. 1998. *Pragmatic Women and Body Politics.* Cambridge: Cambridge University Press.

Lomoro, O. A., J. E. Ehiris, X. Qian, and S. L. Tang. 2002. "Mothers' Perspectives on the Quality of Postpartum Care in Central Shanghai, China," *International Journal for Quality in Health Care* 14:393–401.

Lopez, Iris. 2008. *Matters of Choice: Puerto Rican Women's Struggle for Reproductive Freedom.* New Brunswick, NJ: Rutgers University Press.

Lupton, Deborah. 1995. *The Imperative of Health: Public Health and the Regulated Body.* London: Sage.

Lutsiv, O., E. Pullenayegum, G. Foster, C. Vera, L. Giglia, B. Chapman, C. Fusch, and S. McDonald. 2013a. "A Population-Based Cohort Study of Breastfeeding According to Gestational Age at Term Delivery. *Journal of Pediatrics* 163(5): 1283–88.

Lutsiv O. E. Pullenayegum, G. Foster, C. Vera, L. Giglia, B. Chapman, C. Fusch, and S. McDonald. 2013b, Women's Intentions to Breastfeed: A Population-Based Cohort Study. *British Journal of Obstetrics and Gynecology* 120:1490–99.

Ma, Meiling. 2001. "Nan Zhu Wai, Nu Zhu Nei Xian Xiang Hui Chao" 男主外女主内现象回潮[Men are responsible for public affairs, women are responsible for housework]. *Wen Hui Bao*, November 9.

Maher, Vanessa. 1992. *The Anthropology of Breastfeeding: Natural Law or Social Construct.* Oxford: Berg.

Mahmood, Saba. 2001. "Feminist Theory, Embodiment, and the Docile Agent: Some Reflections on the Egyptian Revival." *Cultural Anthropology* 6(2): 202–36.

Martin, Emily. 1987. *The Woman in the Body: A Cultural Analysis of Reproduction.* Boston: Beacon.

Massey, Doreen. 1993. "Power-Geometry and a Sense of Place." In *Mapping the Futures: Local Cultures, Global Change,* edited by J. Bird, 59–69. London: Routledge.

Masvie, H. 2006. "The Role of Tamang Mothers-in-Law in Promoting Breast Feeding in Makwanpur District, Nepal." *Midwifery* 22:23–31.

McCaughey, Martha. 2010. "Got Milk? Breastfeeding as an 'Incurably Informed' Feminist STS Scholar." *Science as Culture* 19(1): 79–100.

McKenzie, Paul. 1993. "Commentary." *China Law Reporter* 7(1): 7–11.

McLeod, D., S. Pullon, and T. Cookson. 2002. Factors Influencing Continuation of Breastfeeding in a Cohort of Women. *Journal of Human Lactation* 18(4): 335–42.

Mead Johnson Annual Report. 1996.

Melly, Caroline. 2017. *Bottleneck: Moving, Building, and Belonging in an African City.* Chicago: University of Chicago Press.

Meng, Angela. 2014. "China Lifts Ban on Prenatal Genetic Testing." *South China Morning Post,* July 10. http://www.geneticliteracyproject.org/source/south-china-morning-post/

Meng, Xianfan. 1995. *Chinese Women in the Reforms.* Beijing: Chinese Academy of Social Sciences.

Merten, Sonja, Julie Dratva, and Ursula Ackermann-Liebrich. 2005. "Do Baby-Friendly Hospitals Influence Breastfeeding Duration on an International Level?" *Pediatrics* 116:702–8.

Merewood, Anne and Supriya D. Mehta, Laura Beth Chamberlain, Barbara L. Philipp, Howard Bauchner. 2005. "Breastfeeding Rates in US Baby-Friendly Hospitals: Results of a National Survey," *Pediatrics* 113(3): 628–34.

Miller, Daniel. 2012. *Consumption and Its Consequences.* Cambridge, UK: Polity.

Ministry of Health. 1992. *Establishing a Baby-Friendly Hospital* (Jianli Aiying Yiyuan 建立爱婴医院) Ministry of Health Press. Beijing, China.

Mink, Gwendolyn. 1996. *The Wages of Motherhood: Inequality in the Welfare State, 1917–1942.* Ithaca, NY: Cornell University Press.

Mitra, A. K., A. J. Khoury, A. W. Hinton, and C. Carothers. 2004. "Predictors of Breastfeeding Intention among Low-Income Women. *Maternal and Child Health Journal* 8:65–70.

Mohanty, Chandra. 1991. "Introduction-Cartographies of Struggle." In *Third World Women and the Politics of Feminism,* edited by Chandra Mohanty, Ann Russo, and Lourdes Torres, 1–47. Bloomington: Indiana University Press.

Mohanty, Chandra. 2003. *Feminism without Borders: Decolonizing Theory, Practicing Solidarity.* Durham, NC: Duke University Press.

Mok, E., C. Multon, L. Piguel, E. Barroso, V. Goua, P. Christin, M-J. Perez, and R. Hankard. 2008. "Decreased Full Breastfeeding, Altered Practices, Perceptions, and Infant Weight Change in Pre-pregnant Obese Women: A Need for Extra Support." *Pediatrics* 121:1319–24.

Mol, Annemarie, and Eric Berg. 1998. *Differences in Medicine: Unraveling Practices, Techniques, and Bodies.* Durham, NC: Duke University Press.

Molony, Barbara. 1995. "Japan's Equal Opportunity Employment Law and the Changing Discourse on Gender." *Signs: Journal of Women in Culture and Society* 20(2): 268–302.

Morsy, Soheir. 1995. "Deadly Reproduction among Egyptian Women: Maternal Mortality and the Medicalization of Population Control." In *Conceiving the New World Order: The Global Politics of Reproduction,* edited by Faye Ginsburg and Rayna Rapp, 162–76. Berkeley: University of California Press.

Murphy, Michelle. 2012. *Seizing the Means of Reproduction: The Entanglements of Feminism, Health, and Technoscience.* Durham, NC: Duke University Press.

Naylor, Audrey. 1995. "Baby-Friendly Hospital Initiative: Protecting, Promoting, and Supporting Breastfeeding in the Twenty-First Century. *Pediatrics Clinic of North America* 48(2): 475–83.

Nerlove, Sara B. 1974. "Women's Workload and Infant Feeding Practices: A Relationship with Demographic Implications." *Ethnology* 13:207–14.

Notar, Beth. 1994. "Of Labor and Liberation: Images of Women in Current Chinese Television Advertising." *Visual Anthropology Review* 10(2): 29–44.

Notzon, F. C., S. Cnattingius, S. Cole, S. M. Taffel, L. Irgens, and A. K. Daltveit. 1994. "Cesarean Section Delivery in the 1980s: International Comparison by Indication." *American Journal of Obstetrics and Gynecology* 170:495–504.

Obermayer, Carla, and Sarah Castle. 1996. "Back to Nature? Historical and Cross Cultural Perspectives on Barriers to Breastfeeding." *Medical Anthropology* 17(1): 39–63.

O'Donnell, Mary Ann. 2012. "Cat Theory: Contextualizing Deng Xiaoping's Pragmatism," *Shenzhen Noted* (blog), August 22, https://shenzhennoted.com/2012/08/22/cat-theory-contextualizing-deng-xiaopings-pragmatism/

Ong, Aiwha. 1997. "Chinese Modernities: Narratives of Nation and of Capitalism." In *Ungrounded Empires: The Cultural Politics of Modern Chinese Transnationalism,* edited by Donald Nonini and Aiwha Ong, 176-202. New York: Routledge.

Ortner, Sherry. 2006. *Anthropology and Social Theory: Culture, Power, and the Acting Subject.* Durham, NC: Duke University Press.

Osborn, Thomas. 1997. "Of Health and Statecraft." In *Foucault, Health, and Medicine,* edited by Alan Peterson and Robin Bunton, 170–88. New York: Routledge.

Otsuka, Keiko, Masataka Taguri, Cindy-Lee Dennis, Kiriko Wakutani, Masayo Awano, Takuhiro Yamaguchi, and Masamine Jimba. 2013. "Effectiveness of a Breastfeeding Self-Efficacy Intervention: Do Hospital Practices Make a Difference?" *Maternal and Child Health Journal* 18:296–306.

Parker, Lyn, and Laura Dales. 2015. "Introduction: The Everyday Agency of Women." In *Contestations over Gender in Asia,* edited by Lyn Parker, Laura Dales, and Chie Ikeya, 1–23. London: Routledge.

Pasternak, Burton, and Ching Wang. 1985. "Breastfeeding Decline in Urban China: An Exploratory Study." *Human Ecology* 13(4): 433–66.

Paxson, Heather. 2004. *Making Modern Mothers: Ethics and Family Planning in Urban Greece.* Berkeley: University of California Press.

Petersen, Alan. 1997. "Risk, Governance, and the New Public Health." In *Foucault, Health, and Medicine,* edited by Alan Petersen and Robin Bunton, 189–206. New York: Routledge.

Petersen, Alan, and Deborah Lupton. 1997. *The New Public Health: Health and Self in the Age of Risk.* London: Sage.

Phillip, Barbara and Anne Merewood. 2004. "The Baby-Friendly Way: The Best Breastfeeding Start." Pediatric Clinics of North America 51(3): 761-783.

Pillsbury, Barbara. 1978. "'Doing the Month': Confinement and Convalescence of Chinese Women after Childbirth." *Social Science and Medicine* 12:11–22.

Piperata, Barbara A., and Darna L. Dufour. 2007. "Diet, Energy Expenditure, and Body Composition of Lactating Ribeirinha Women in the Brazilian Amazon." *American Journal of Human Biology* 19(5): 722–34.

Popkin, B. R., J. Bilsborrow, J. Akin, and M. Yamamato. 1986. "Breastfeeding Determinants in Low Income Countries." *Family Planning* 9:1–31.

Proffitt, Allison. 2013. "Fruitful Market: Berry Genomics Tackles Prenatal Testing in China." *Bio-It World.* http://www.bio-itworld.com/2013/2/20/fruitful-market-berry-genomics-tackles-prenatal-testing-china.html

Putterman, Louis, and Xiaoyuan Dong. 2002. "China's State-Owned Enterprises in the First Reform Decade: An Analysis of a Declining Monopsony." *Economics of Planning* 35(2): 109–40.

Qian Xu, Helen Smith, Li Zhou, Ji Liang, and Paul Gartner. 2001. "Evidence-Based Obstetrics in Four Hospitals in China: An Observational Study to Explore Clinical Practice, Women's Preferences, and Provider Views." *BMC Pregnancy and Childbirth* 2001: 1(1), doi: 10.1186/1471-2393-1-1.

Qiu, Liqian, Colin Binns, Yun Zhao, Andy H. Lee, and Xing Xie. 2010. "Breastfeeding Practice in Zhejiang Province, PR China, in the Context of Melamine-Contaminated Formula Milk." *Journal of Health Population and Nutrition* 28(2): 189–98.

Quandt, Sarah. 1995. "Sociocultural Aspects of the Lactation Process." In *Breastfeeding: Biocultural Perspectives,* edited by Patricia Stuart Macadam and Katherine Detwyler, 128–44. New York: Aldine de Gruyter.

Rabinow, Paul and Nikolas Rose. 2006. "Biopower Today." *Biosocieties* 1: 195–217.

Ram, Kalpana, and Margaret Jolly, eds. 1998. *Maternities and Modernities: Colonial and Post-colonial Experiences in Asia and the Pacific.* Cambridge: Cambridge University Press.

Riley, Nancy. 1996. "Holding Up Half the Economy." *China Business Review* 23(1): 8–17.

Rivkin-Fish, Michele. 2005. *Women's Health in Post-Soviet Russia: The Politics of Intervention.* Bloomington: Indiana University Press.

Robinson, Jean C. 1985. "Of Women and Washing Machines: Employment, Housework, and the Reproduction of Motherhood in Socialist China." *China Quarterly* 3(101): 32–57.

Rofel, Lisa. 1999. *Other Modernities: Gendered Yearnings in China after Socialism.* Berkeley: University of California Press.

Rofel, Lisa. 2007. *Desiring China: Experiments in Neoliberalism, Sexuality, and Public Culture.* Durham, NC: Duke University Press.

Rose, Nikolas. 2007. *The Politics of Life Itself: Biomedicine, Power, and Subjectivity in the Twenty-First Century.* Princeton, NJ: Princeton University Press.

Rosenberg K. D., J. D. Stull, and M. R. Adler. 2008. "Impact of Hospital Policies on Breastfeeding Outcomes." *Breastfeeding Medicine* 3:110–16.

Rothman Barbara Katz. 1991. *Recreating Motherhood: Ideology and Technology in a Patriarchal Society.* New York: Norton.

Rudzik, Alanna E. F. 2012. "The Experience and Determinants of First-Time Breast-Feeding Duration among Low-Income Women from Sao Paulo, Brazil." *Current Anthropology* 53(1): 108–17.

Santos, Goncalo. 2006. "The Anthropology of Chinese Kinship: A Critical Overview." *European Journal of East Asian Studies* 5(2): 275–333.

Sargent, Carolyn and Nancy Stark. 1988. "Childbirth Education and Childbirth Models: Parental Perspectives on Control, Anesthesia, and Technological Intervention in the Birth Process." *Medical Anthropology Quarterly* 3(1): 36–51.

Schein, Louisa. 1999. "Of Cargo and Satellites: Imagined Cosmopolitanism." *Postcolonial Studies* 2(3): 345–75.

Scheper-Hughes, Nancy. 1984. "Infant Mortality and Infant Care: Cultural and Economic Constraints on Nurturing in Northeast Brazil." *Social Science and Medicine* 19(5): 535–46.

Scheper-Hughes, Nancy. 1987. *Child Survival: Anthropological Perspectives on the Treatment and Maltreatment of Children.* Dordrecht: Kluwer.

Scheper-Hughes, Nancy. 1992. *Death without Weeping: The Violence of Everyday Life in Brazil.* Berkeley: University of California Press.

Scheper-Hughes, Nancy, and Margaret Lock. 1987. "The Mindful Body: A Prolegomenon to Future Work in Medical Anthropology." *Medical Anthropology Quarterly* 1(1): 6–41.

Shanghai Educational Television. 1994. *Muru Weiyang*母乳喂养 *Breastfeeding.* Video recording.

Shaw, Rhonda and Alison Bartlett. 2010. *Giving Breastmilk: Body Ethics and Contemporary Breastfeeding Practices.* New South Wales, Australia: University of New South Wales.

Short, Susan, Feinian Chen, Barbara Entwistle, and Zhai Fengying. 2002. "Maternal Work and Time Spent in Child Care in China: A Multimethod Approach." *Population and Development Review* 28(1): 31–57.

Siti, Aisyah and Lyn Parker. 2014. "Problematic Conjugations: Women's Agency, Marriage, and Domestic Violence in Indonesia." *Asian Studies Review* 38(2): 205-223.

Sleeboom-Faulkner, Margaret. 2010. "Eugenic Birth and Fetal Education: The Friction between Lineage Enhancement and Premarital Testing among Rural Households in Mainland China." *China Journal* 64:121–41.

Solinger, Dorothy. 1999. *Contesting Citizenship in Urban China: Peasant Migrants, the State, and the Logic of Market.* Berkeley: University of California Press.

Stacey, Jackie. 2000. "The Global Within: Consuming Nature, Embodying Health." In *Global Nature Global Culture,* edited by Sarah Franklin, Celia Lury, and Jackie Stacey, 97–144. Thousand Oaks, CA: Sage.

Stacey, Judith. 1983. *Patriarchy and the Socialist Revolution in China.* Berkeley: University of California Press.

Stack, Carol, and Linda Burton. 1994. "Kinscripts: Reflections on Family, Generation, and Culture." In *Mothering: Ideology, Experience, and Agency,* edited by Evelyn Nakano Glenn, Grace Chang, and Linda Rennie Forcey, 33–44. New York: Routledge.

State of Israel Ministry of Trade. 2012. "Cosmetics Giants Brush Off Any Talk of Slump in China." State of Israel Ministry of Trade, November 27. http://itrade.gov.il/china-en/2012/11/27/cosmetics-giants-brush-off-any-talk-of-slump-in-china//#sthash.hLdF5Epd.dpuf

Stearns Cindy. 2013. "The Embodied Practices of Breastfeeding: Implications for Research and Policy." *Journal of Women, Politics, and Policy* 34(4): 359–70.

Steinberg, Suzanne. 1996. "Childbearing Research: A Transcultural View." *Social Science and Medicine* 43(12): 1765–84.

Stevenson-Yang, Anne. 1996. "Revamping the Welfare State." *China Business Review* 32(1): 822–24.

Stoss, Randall. 1988. "The Return of Advertising in China: A Study of the Ideological Reversal." *China Quarterly* 123:485–502.

Strathern, Andrew. 1996. *Body Thoughts.* Ann Arbor: University of Michigan Press.

Su Haiying. 1997. "'Reassured Egg' Boiled by Mother in Law: An Anthropologic Investigation on the Lying in of Han Women in the Three Gorges Area." *Journal of the South West Institute for Ethnic Groups* 1:22–26.

Sun Wen Li. 2011. "Distribution of Free Formula in Hospitals: The Regulation Is Violated." *Peninsula City News,* November 2. In Chinese. Accessed April 22, 2014. http://qingdao.dzwww.com/xinwen/qingdaonews/201111/t20111102_6737719.htm

Sun Zhongxin. 2008. "Worker, Woman, Mother: Redefining Urban Chinese Women's Identity via Motherhood and the Global Workplace." *Asian Journal of Women's Studies* 14(1): 7–35.

Swanson, Mitzie. 1995. "China Puts on a New Face." *China Business Review* 22(5): 34–36.

Tang, L., A. H. Lee, C. W. Binns, Y. Yang, Y. Wu, Y. Li, and L. Qiu. 2014. "Widespread Usage of Infant Formula in China: A Major Public Health Problem." *Birth* 41(4): 339–43.

Tarrant, Marie, Kendra Wu, Daniel Fong, Irene Lee, Emmy Wong, Alice Sham, Christine Lam, and Joan Dodgson. 2011. "Impact of Baby-Friendly Hospital Practices on Breastfeeding in Hong Kong." *Birth* 38(3): 238–45.

Taussig, Karen-Sue, Klaus Hoeyer, and Stefan Helmreich. 2013. "The Anthropology of Potentiality in Biomedicine: An Introduction to Supplement 7." *Current Anthropology* 54(suppl. 7): S3–14.

Taylor, Janelle. 2004. "Introduction." In *Consuming Motherhood,* edited by Janelle Taylor, Linda Layne, and Danielle F. Wozniak, 1–18. New Brunswick, NJ: Rutgers University Press.

Teman, Elly. 2009. Embodying Surrogate Motherhood: Pregnancy as a Dyadic Body Project. *Body and Society* 15(3): 47-69.

Teman, Elly, Tsipy Ivry, and Heela Goren. 2016. "Hishtadlut [Obligatory Effort] as an Explanatory Model: A Critique of Reproductive Choice and Control." *Culture Medicine and Psychiatry* 40(2): 268–88.

Tomba, Luigi. 2009. "Of Quality, Harmony, and Community: Civilization and the Middle Class in Urban China." *positions: east asia cultures critique* 17(3): 591–616.

Tong, Xin. 2010. "Mainstream Discourse and the Construction of Public Understanding of Women's Employment." *Social Sciences in China* 31(2): 135–49.

Topley, Marjorie. 1976. "Chinese Traditional Etiology and Methods of Cure in Hong Kong." In *Asian Medical Systems: A Comparative Study,* edited by Charles Leslie, 243–65. Berkeley: University of California Press.

Trussell J., L. Grummer-Strawn, G. Rodriguez, and M. Van Landingham. 1992. "Trends and Differentials in Breastfeeding Behaviour: Evidence from the WFS and DHS." *Population Studies* 46(2): 285–307.

Tsing, Anna Lowenhaupt. 2004. *Friction: An Ethnography of Global Connection.* Princeton, NJ: Princeton University Press.

Turner, Terence. 1994. "Bodies and Anti-bodies: Flesh and Fetish in Contemporary Social Theory." *In Embodiment and Experience: The Existential Ground of Culture and Self,* edited by Thomas Csordas, 27–47. Cambridge: Cambridge University Press.

UNICEF. 2005. *The Baby Friendly Hospital Initiative,* January 1, 2005. Accessed May 25, 2016. https://www.unicef.org/nutrition/index_24806.html

UNICEF. 2007. *Infant and Young Child Feeding and Care.* Accessed March 13, 2008. http://www.unicef.org/nutrition/index_24819.html

UNICEF/WHO. 1996. "The Challenge to Nature." Pamphlet.

United Nations. 1995. *Baby Friendly Hospital Initiative Newsletter* 5:1.

United Nations. 1996. *Baby Friendly Hospital Initiative Newsletter* 7:3.

Unnithan-Kumar, Maya. 2004. "Introduction." In *Reproductive Agency, Medicine, and the State: Cultural Transformations in Childbearing*, edited by Maya Unnithan-Kumar, 1–24. New York: Berghahn.

Van Esterik, Penny. 1989. *Beyond the Breast-Bottle Controversy*. New Brunswick, NJ: Rutgers University Press.

Van Esterik, Penny. 1995a. "Care, Caregiving, and Caregivers." *Food and Nutrition Bulletin* 16(4): 378–88.

Van Esterik, Penny. 1995b. "The Politics of Breastfeeding: An Advocacy Perspective." In *Breastfeeding: Biocultural Perspectives,* edited by Patricia Stuart Macadam and Katherine Detwyler, 145–66. New York: Aldine de Gruyter.

Van Esterik, Penny. 2004. "Contemporary Trends in Infant Feeding Research." *Annual Review of Anthropology* 31:257–58.

Van Hollen, Cecilia. 2003. *Birth on the Threshold: Childbirth and Modernity in South India*. Berkeley: University of California Press.

Van Hollen, Cecilia. 2011. "Breast or Bottle? HIV-Positive Women's Responses to Global Health Policy on Infant Feeding in India." *Medical Anthropology Quarterly* 25(4): 499–518.

Van Wolputte, Steven. 2004. "Hang on to Your Self: Of Bodies, Embodiment, and Selves. *Annual Review of Anthropology* 33:251–69.

Vogel, Suzanne. 1996. "Urban Middle Class Japanese Family Life, 1958–1996: A Personal and Evolving Perspective." In *Japanese Childrearing: Two Generations of Scholarship,* edited by David Shwalb and Barbara Shwalb, 177–200. New York: Guilford.

Wall, Glenda. 2001. "Moral Constructions of Motherhood in Breastfeeding Discourse." *Gender and Society* 15(4): 592–610.

Wallis, Cara. 2013. *Technomobility in China: Young Migrant Women and Mobile Phones*. New York: New York University Press.

Wang, Aihua. 1994. *Renshen yu fenmian da quan* 妊娠与分娩大全 [The complete book of pregnancy and birth]. Zhongshan: Zhongshan Chubenshe.

Wang Xiaoli, Yan Wang, and Sui Zhou. 2009. "The Relationship between Taboos and Chronic Pain in Postpartum Women in Rural Areas." *Maternal and Child Health Care of China*, 2009:23. http://en.cnki.com.cn/Article_en/CJFDTOTAL-ZFYB200923041.htm

Wang Xiaoli, Yan Wang, Sui Zanzhou, Jing Wang, and Jianlin Wang. 2008. A Population-Based Survey of Women's Traditional Postpartum Behaviors in Northern China. *Midwifery* 24:238–45.

Wang, Zheng. 2003. "Gender, Employment, and Women's Resistance." In *Chinese Society, Change, Conflict, and Resistance,* edited by Liz Perry and Mark Selden, 138–82. New York: Routledge Curzon.

Watson, Rubie S., and Patricia Ebrey. 1989. *Marriage and Inequality in Chinese Society*. Berkeley University of California Press.

Wei Luo. 2013. "Aching for the Altered Body: Beauty Economy and Chinese Women's Consumption of Cosmetic Surgery." *Women's Studies International Forum* 38(3): 1–10.

Wilmoth, Teresa A., and John P. Elder. 1995. "An Assessment of Research on Breastfeeding Promotion Strategies in Developing Countries." *Social Science and Medicine* 41(4): 579–94.

Winkler, Edward A. 2005. "Maximizing the Impact of Cairo on China." In *Where Human Rights Begin: Essays on Health, Sexuality, and Women Ten Years after Vienna, Cairo, and Beijing,* edited by Wendy Chavkin and Ellen Chesler, 204–34. Piscataway, NJ: Rutgers University Press.

Wolf, Joan. 2010. *Is Breast Best? Taking on the Breastfeeding Experts and the New High Stakes of Motherhood.* New York: New York University Press.

Wolf, Margery. 1978. *Women and the Family in Rural Taiwan.* Palo Alto, CA: Stanford University Press.

Wolf, Margery. 1985. *Revolution Postponed: Women in Contemporary China.* Palo Alto, CA: Stanford University Press.

Woo, Margaret. 1993. "Biology and Equality: Challenges for Feminism in the Socialist and Liberal State." *Emory Law Journal* 4(1): 143–96.

World Health Organization. 1981. "Innocenti Declaration." https://www.unicef.org/programme/breastfeeding/innocenti.htm

World Health Organization. 1986. "The Ottawa Charter for Health Promotion." First International Conference on Health Promotion, Ottawa, November 21.

World Health Organization. 2000. "World Health Organization Collaborative Study Team on the Role of Breastfeeding in the Prevention of Infant Mortality: effect of breastfeeding on infant and child mortality due to infectious diseases in less developed countries: a pooled analysis." *Lancet* 355: 451–55.

World Health Organization. 2007. *Care in Normal Birth: A Practical Guide.* Geneva: World Health Organization. Report of a Technical Working Group.

Wu, Kangmin, Renwei Dong, Weiguang Xu, Yucheng Xun, and Liu Qing. 1995. "Chengdu Shi Qu Muru Weiyang Xian Zhuang Jiqi Yingxiang Yinsu Diaocha." 成都市区母乳喂养现状激起影响因素调查 (Investigation of Factors Influencing Breastfeeding in Urban Chengdu) *Hua Xi Yi Xue* 10(2): 174–76.

Wu, Wangling. 2000. "Cesarean Delivery in Shantou China: A Retrospective Analysis of 1,922 Women." *Birth* 27(2): 86–90.

Wu, Xiaoying. 2010. "From State Dominance to Market Orientation: The Composition and Evolution of Gender Discourse." *Social Sciences in China* 31(2): 150–64.

Wu Yuxao and Zhou Dongyang. 2015. "Women's Labor Force Participation in Urban China, 1990–2010." *Chinese Sociological Review* 47(4): 314–42.

Xie, Jili. 1992. "Youguan Muru Weiyang de Xin Guandian." 有关母乳喂养的新观点(New Ideas about Breastfeeding) *Hushi Jinxiu Zazhi* 7(1): 10–11.

Xinhua News Agency. 1995. "Maternal and Infant Welfare Law." *Foreign Broadcast Information Services,* November 21.

Xinhua News Agency 1996a. "Beijing Issues Child Welfare White Paper." *Foreign Broadcast Information Services,* December 9.

Xinhua News Agency 1996b. "China Leads in Baby-Friendly Hospital Initiative." *Foreign Broadcast Information Services,* April 3.

Xinhua News Agency. 1996c. "The Situation of Children in China." April 3.

Xu, Fuqi. 1929. "Preface," *Niuru Yanjiu (Milk Research) Minzhi Shuji.* In Susan Glosser, "Milk for Health, Milk for Profit: Shanghai's Chinese Dairy Industry under Japanese Occupation." In *Inventing Nanjing Road: Commercial Culture in Shanghai, 1900–1945,* edited by Sherman Cochran, 207–33. East Asia Series. Ithaca, NY: Cornell University Press, 1999.

Xun, Zhongyong, Lu Xiuping, Li Qinghua, Zhou Mei, Wang Yongqin, and Yan Bufan. 1995. "Cheng Xiang Muru Weiyang Ji Muru Xiguan Diaocha."城乡母乳喂养己母乳习惯调查[Survey of Breastfeeding Preferences in Urban and Rural Areas] *Weifang Yixue Yuanxue Bao* 17(3): 207–8.

Yan, Yunxiang. 2003. *Private Life under Socialism: Love, Intimacy, and Family Change in a Chinese Village, 1949–1999.* Palo Alto, CA: Stanford University Press.

Yan, Yunxiang. 2009. "The Good Samaritan's New Trouble: A Study of the Changing Moral Landscape in Contemporary China." *Social Anthropology* 17(1): 9–24.

Yan, Yunxiang. 2011. "The Individualization of the Family in Rural China." *boundary 2* 38(1): 203–29.

Yang, Jie. 2011. "Nennu and Shunu: Gender, Body Politics, and the Beauty Economy in China." *Signs: Journal of Women in Culture and Society* 36(2): 333–57.

Yang, P. Y., Z. S. Kang, L. J. Ling, and Q. C. Xin. 1989. "Breastfeeding of Infants between 0–6 Months in 20 Provinces, Municipalities, and Autonomous Regions in the People's Republic of China." *Journal of Tropical Pediatrics* 35:277–80.

Yang, Youde, 1992. *Huai Chan Cu Jianshen Bao Tai 500 Zhao.* 坏产促健身保胎500找 *(Prevent Miscarriage by Watching for These 500 Urgent Problems During Pregnancy).* Tianjin: Tianjin Keji Chubenshe.

Yang, Zhenyu, Lai Jianqing, Yu Dongmei, Yifan Duan, Xuehong Pang, Shan Jiang, Ye Bi, Jie Wang, Liyun Zhao, and Shian Yin. 2016. "Breastfeeding Rates in China: A Cross-Sectional Survey and Estimate of Benefits of Improvement." The *Lancet,* 388:S47. Accessed February 22, 2017. http://dx.doi.org/10.1016/S0140-6736(16)31974-2

Yuan, Xiaohong. 1997. "Baby-Friendly Action in China: Protection, Promotion, and Support of Breastfeeding." In *1997 Asian Conference of Pediatricians Abstracts.*

Zadoroznyj, Maria. 2001. "Birth and the 'Reflexive Consumer': Trust, Risk and Medical Dominance in Obstetrical Encounters." *Journal of Sociology* 37(2): 117–39.

Zha, Jianying. 1995. *China Pop.* New York: New Press.

Zhang, Li. 2010. *In Search of Paradise: Middle Class Living in a Chinese Metropolis.* Ithaca, NY: Cornell University Press.

Zhang Li and Aihwa Ong. 2008. *Privatizing China: Socialism from Afar.* Ithaca, NY: Cornell University Press.

Zhang, Tony Huiquan, Robert Brym, and Robert Anderson. 2017. "Liberalism and Postmaterialism in China: The Role of Social Class and Inequality." *Chinese Sociological Review* 49(1): 65–87.

Zhao Dan. 2014. "Yuezi Zhongxin Zuo Yuezi Zui Gui Ershi Wan" 月子中心做月子最贵二十万 [Most expensive sitting the month center now ¥200,000]. *Dong Fang Ribao,* May 24. Accessed June 2015. http://wenku.baidu.com/view/a7adbb4e4431b90d6d85c713.html

Zhao Suisheng. 1993. "Deng Xiaoping's Southern Tour: Elite Politics in Post-Tiananmen China." *Asian Survey* 33(8): 739–56.

Zhao Xu, Yining Peng, and Yang Yang. 2013. "Bribery Claims Feed Milk Scandal." *China Daily,* 22 October. Accessed April 22, 2014. http://usa.chinadaily.com.cn/china/2013-10/22/content_17049396.htm

Zhao, Y., A. M. Niu, G. F. Xu, M. J. Garrett, and T. Greiner. 2003. "Early Infant Feeding Practices in Jinan City, Shandong Province, China." *Asia Journal of Clinical Nutrition* 12(1): 104–8.

Zheng, Tiantian. 2009. *Red Lights: The Lives of Sex Workers in Postsocialist China.* Minneapolis: University of Minnesota Press.

Zheng, Zhihua. 1992. "Chengshi Nianqing Funu Xiaofei Wuqu城市年青妇女消费误" [Urban young women's mistaken ideas consumption]. *Zhonguo Shehui Bao* 4(10): 4.

Zhu, Baoxia. 1994. "Breast-Feed Babies, Says Conference." *China Daily,* July 30, 3.

Zhu Jianfeng. 2010. "Mothering Expectant Mothers: Consumption, Production, and Two Motherhoods in Contemporary China." *Ethos* 38(4): 406–12.

Zhu Jianfeng. 2013. "Projecting Potentiality: Understanding Maternal Serum Screening in Contemporary China." *Current Anthropology* 54(suppl. 7): S36–44.

Zhu Jianfeng. 2016. "Understanding the Cradle Project: Fetal Education, Modern Cerebral Science, and Traditional Chinese Medical Practice in Contemporary China." Paper presented at the Society for the History of Technology, Singapore, June 23.

Zhu, Sophia. 2014. "Hit TV Show Reflects Parents' Anxiety." Women of China January 7. http://www.womenofchina.cn/womenofchina/html1/opinion/16/8728-1.htm

Index